DONNA ATTARD

Toxin Free Eco Baby

Copyright © 2024 by Donna Attard

All rights reserved. No part of this publication may be reproduced, stored or transmitted in any form or by any means, electronic, mechanical, photocopying, recording, scanning, or otherwise without written permission from the publisher. It is illegal to copy this book, post it to a website, or distribute it by any other means without permission.

Donna Attard has no responsibility for the persistence or accuracy of URLs for external or third-party Internet Websites referred to in this publication and does not guarantee that any content on such Websites is, or will remain, accurate or appropriate.

The information provided in this book, "Toxin Free Eco Baby: How to Create a Healthy & Chemical Free Home for Your Little One' is intended for educational and informational purposes only. While every effort has been made to ensure the accuracy and reliability of the content, the author and publisher make no representations or warranties of any kind, express or implied, about the completeness, accuracy, reliability, suitability, or availability with respect to the book's content.

The recommendations and advice offered are based on personal experiences and research, and they may not be suitable for every individual or situation. Readers are encouraged to consult with healthcare professionals, environmental experts, and other qualified advisors to determine the best practices for their specific circumstances. The reader assumes full responsibility for his or her own actions and decisions regarding their health, their baby's health and non-toxic living.

First edition

This book was professionally typeset on Reedsy.
Find out more at reedsy.com

Your Non Toxic Eco Baby

Amid the fast-paced world of modern parenthood, a gentle revolution is taking place – parents of today are shifting toward a more conscious and healthy way of nurturing their children.

Welcome to a new chapter in your parenting journey, where creating a non toxic and healthy home for your baby is both a commitment and a necessity. In Toxin Free Eco Baby: How to Create a Healthy & Chemical Free Home for Your Little One, we will explore simple ways to make conscious choices that benefit you and your baby's wellbeing, as well as supporting the nourishment of our planet, as our children are the future guardians of earth and all who live upon her.

From sustainable baby gear and personal care products, to eco friendly nursery set-ups, to chemical-free daily practices, allow me to guide you through practical steps and inspiring ideas to love and nurture your baby in a safe and healthy home. Together, let's embark on this exciting path to raise a new generation of children that are strong and happy, are nutritionally nourished and that respect and protect the earth.

Raising a toxin-free baby starts with simple decisions that gradually evolve into a lifestyle centred around safe and healthy choices for both you and your family.

Tips for a Healthy Home

Bringing your little one into a toxin free and healthy home is the ultimate welcome for your baby.

Choose Non-Toxic Paints and Materials:
Use non-toxic, low-VOC paint for the nursery and throughout the home. Choose eco-friendly and chemical free building materials and finishes whenever possible to reduce exposure to harmful chemicals.

Create a Sustainable Nursery:
Furnish the nursery with sustainable and non-toxic furniture made from materials such as bamboo, reclaimed wood, or FSC-certified (Forest Stewardship Council) wood. Use organic bedding, non synthetic crib mattresses and natural textiles to provide a safe and healthy sleeping environment for your baby.

Use Natural and Organic Baby Products:
Choose natural and organic baby care products, including skincare, diapers, wipes and laundry detergent. Look for products with minimal packaging and eco-friendly certifications to reduce waste and minimise environmental impact.

Cloth Diapers (Nappies):
Consider using cloth diapers instead of disposable diapers to reduce waste and save money in the long run. Cloth diapers are available in a variety of styles and materials, including organic cotton, bamboo and hemp.

Breastfeed if Possible:
Breastfeeding is not only beneficial for your baby's health but also environmentally friendly, as it reduces the need for formula production and packaging. If breastfeeding is not an option, choose an organic formula packaged in eco-friendly materials.

Practice Waste Reduction:

Reduce waste by using reusable products such as cloth wipes, nursing pads and glass or stainless steel baby bottles. Minimise single-use plastics and opt for reusable alternatives such as stainless steel or silicone food containers, water bottles and snack bags.

Energy Efficiency:

Invest in energy-efficient appliances and use natural lighting whenever possible. Install blackout curtains or shades in the nursery to help your baby sleep.

Green Cleaning:

Clean your home with eco-friendly cleaning products made from natural ingredients such as vinegar, baking soda and essential oils. Avoid harsh chemicals and synthetic fragrances and perfumes, often found in everyday cleaning products, that can be harmful to your baby's health.

Connect with Nature:

Spend time outdoors with your baby, exploring nature and connecting with the natural world. Take nature walks, visit parks and gardens and cultivate a love and appreciation for the environment together as a family.

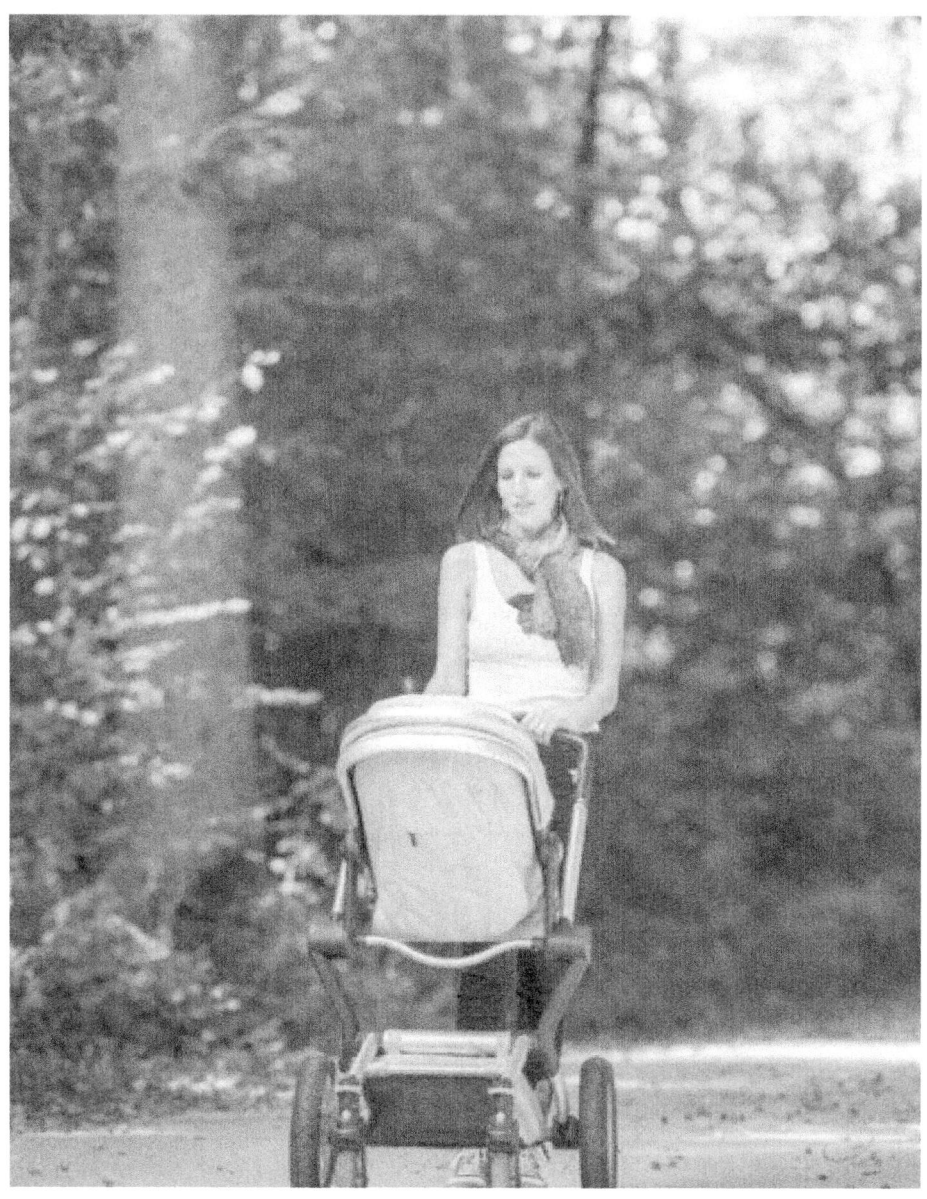

Why Chemical-Free Parenting Matters

Being a chemical-free parent directly impacts the wellbeing of your baby, the health of the environment, and the future of our society as a whole. Chemical-free parenting is a holistic approach that encompasses environmental, health, financial, educational, and social aspects. By adopting eco-sustainable practices you, as a parent, can significantly contribute to the wellbeing of your children, the preservation of nature and the creation of a more responsible and sustainable society.

Health Benefits

Reducing your baby's exposure to toxic chemicals, such as chemically-laden pesticides and fertilisers, through using organic and locally sourced foods, can positively impact your baby's development and growth.

Environmental Impact

Teaching your children to value and conserve resources helps reduce waste and lowers the overall consumption of natural resources. Sustainable practices, such as using reusable products and reducing energy consumption, contribute to lowering your family's carbon footprint. Choosing eco friendly, non toxic products and reducing the use of harmful chemicals helps minimise pollution and protects natural ecosystems.

Financial Savings

Sustainable choices, such as buying second-hand items, using cloth diapers, and reducing energy consumption, can lead to significant financial savings over time.

Community and Social Impact

Participating in community gardens, local clean-up efforts, and other environmental initiatives strengthens community bonds and promotes collective action. Teaching your children about social justice issues related to environmental sustainability fosters empathy and a sense of responsibility toward others and the planet.

Long-Term Wellbeing

Chemical-free parenting helps your child to grow up healthy and happy, with the knowledge and habits needed to live sustainably, encouraging your children to prioritise and protect their own health and the health of their surrounding environment.

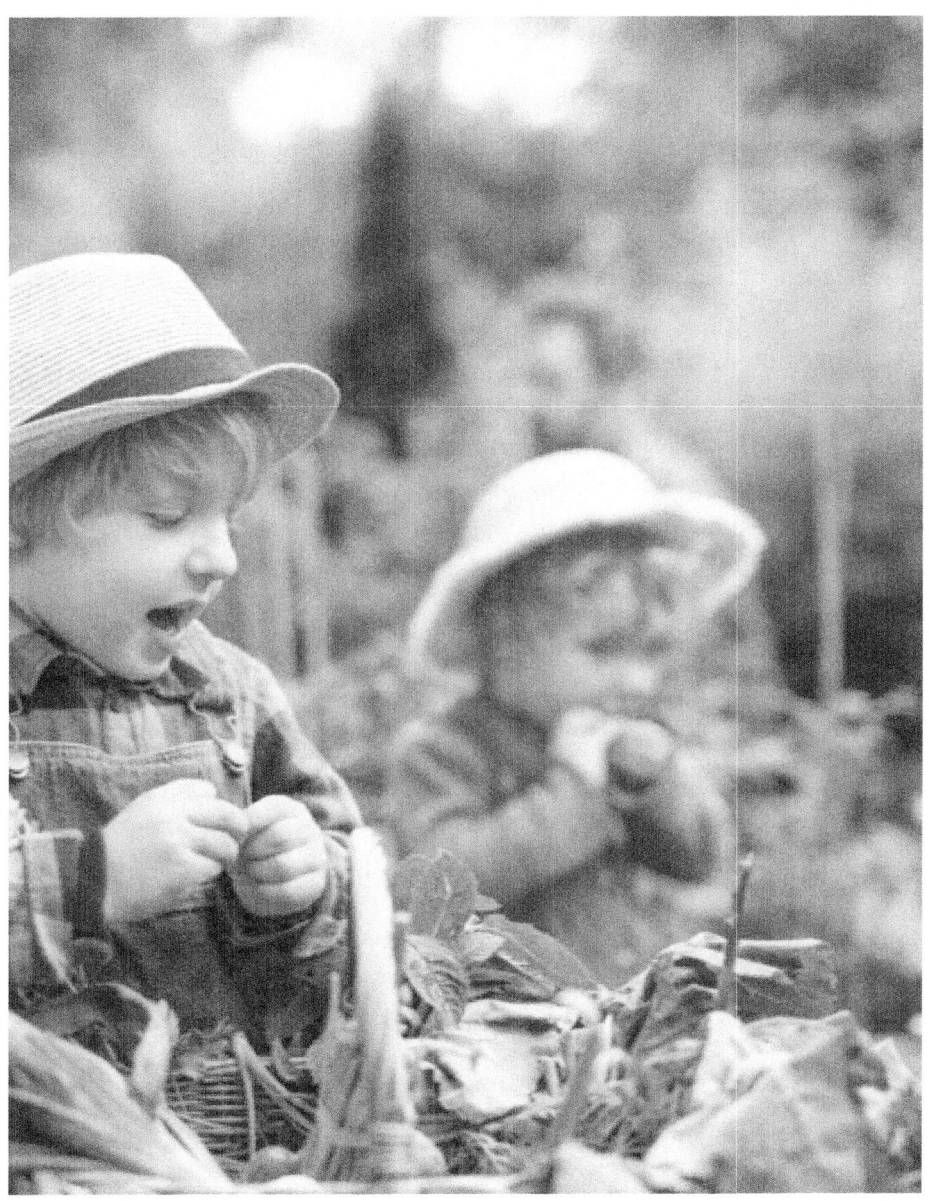

Creating a Toxin Free Nursery for Your Baby

Every decision you make for your baby's nursery, from the materials used in furniture to the products chosen for your baby's bedding, offers a host of benefits that extend far beyond the confines of the nursery walls. By embracing a toxin free approach, you not only safeguard your child's and your family's health and comfort, but also plays a vital role in conserving natural resources.

Healthier Indoor Air Quality

Using paint, furniture, and flooring that are free from volatile organic compounds (VOCs) reduces the presence of harmful chemicals in the air. Organic cotton, wool and other natural fibres in bedding, curtains and clothing minimise exposure to synthetic chemicals and the off-gassing of toxic compounds into the air in baby's nursery.

Reduced Exposure to Toxins

Choosing furniture with non-toxic finishes and adhesives reduces your baby's exposure to harmful substances. By using natural and eco friendly baby care and cleaning products also reduces the risk of respiratory issues and skin irritations for your baby.

Contact with Baby's Skin

Natural materials for baby's clothing and bedding, such as organic cotton, wool and bamboo, are typically free from harmful chemicals and synthetic additives, reducing the risk of further exposure to toxins that can cause allergies or other health issues. Natural fibres tend to be softer and more comfortable against baby's skin, providing a soothing and cosy environment that can contribute to better sleep and overall wellbeing.

Enhanced Comfort and Safety

Natural, breathable fibres are better at regulating body temperature, keeping your baby warm in cooler weather and cool in warmer weather, thereby enhancing your baby's comfort and reducing the risk of overheating.

Ergonomic Design

Eco-friendly furniture often emphasises ergonomic design, providing better support and comfort for both you and your baby.

Cost Savings

Eco friendly products are often more durable, longer lasting and of higher quality, leading to long-term savings.

Promotes Sustainable Practices

Creating an eco friendly nursery encourages a mindset of mindful purchasing and sustainability, setting a positive example for your child as they grow.

Reduced Waste

By choosing reusable and recyclable furniture and other baby products, you contribute to reducing waste and minimising your environmental footprint.

Support for Green Companies

Purchasing from eco friendly brands supports businesses that prioritise family health, toxin free living and environmental responsibility.

Peace of Mind

Knowing that you are making choices that are beneficial for your baby, your family and the planet, can give peace of mind and a sense of personal fulfillment.

Toxin Free Nursery Furniture

Choosing safe and sustainable furniture for your baby's nursery involves selecting pieces that are made from healthy, non toxic materials, renewable resources and are produced and manufactured in an environmentally responsible manner. There are several key factors to consider when purchasing furniture for your baby's room.

Furniture Materials:
  Solid Wood:
  Choose solid wood furniture, preferably sourced from sustainably managed forests (FSC certification).
  Bamboo:
  A rapidly renewable resource that is durable and eco-friendly.
  Recycled Materials:
  Furniture made from recycled or upcycled materials.

Non-Toxic Finishes:
  Ensure that paints, stains, and finishes are non toxic and low-VOC or zero-VOC.

Durability:
  Choose high-quality, durable furniture that can grow with your child or be reused by future siblings, thus reducing waste. Many eco cribs convert into toddler beds, and then into full size adult beds.

Multi-Functional Pieces:
  Furniture that serves multiple purposes, such as convertible cribs or dressers that can be used as changing tables, helps reduce the need for additional pieces.

Certifications:

Look for certifications like GREENGUARD Gold, which ensures that the furniture has low chemical emissions and contributes to healthier indoor air quality.

UL GREENGUARD Gold Certification

The UL GREENGUARD Gold Certification Standard includes health-based criteria for additional chemicals and also requires lower total VOC emission levels.

In addition to limiting emissions of more than 360 VOCs and total chemical emissions, UL GREENGUARD Gold Certified products must also comply with requirements of the state of California Department of Public Health (CDPH) Standard Method for the Testing and Evaluation of Volatile Organic Chemical Emissions from Indoor Sources Using Environmental Chambers, also known as California Section 01350.

All certified products are subject to a review of the manufacturing process and routine testing to minimise impact on the indoor environment.

GECA (Good Environmental Choice Australia)

In Australia, the equivalent certification to the UL GREENGUARD Gold Certification is the GECA (Good Environmental Choice Australia) certification. GECA certification ensures that products meet rigorous standards for low chemical emissions and environmental impact, similar to the criteria used by UL GREENGUARD Gold. GECA-certified products are evaluated for their impact on indoor air quality, making them a reliable choice for creating a safe and healthy environment, such as in a baby's nursery.

What are Volatile Organic Compounds (VOC's)

The majority of everyday chemical exposure in people occurs through the air we breathe in our homes, offices, schools and other indoor environments. These airborne chemicals are commonly referred to as volatile organic compounds (VOCs), used to manufacture and maintain building materials, interior furnishing, cleaning products and personal care products. The U.S. Environmental Protection Agency (EPA) and other researchers have conducted studies and found that VOCs are common in indoor environments and that their levels may be two to a thousand times higher than the air outdoors.

Volatile Organic Compounds (VOCs) are chemicals that easily evaporate into the air at room temperature. They are found in many household products, including paints, adhesives, and furniture made from particle board and MDF.

VOCs can cause health problems such as headaches, dizziness, respiratory issues and eye irritation. In a baby's nursery, exposure to VOCs should be avoided because infants are more sensitive to these chemicals, which can impact their development and overall health.

Using VOC-free materials helps ensure a safer and healthier environment for your baby.

Hidden VOC Hazards in Nursery Furniture

Formaldehyde: Both particle board and MDF often use urea-formaldehyde (UF) resins as a binding agent. Formaldehyde is a known carcinogen and can off-gas into the indoor environment, causing respiratory issues, eye irritation and other health problems.

Volatile Organic Compounds (VOCs): In addition to formaldehyde, these materials can emit other VOCs, which contribute to indoor air pollution and can cause headaches, dizziness and long-term health issues.

Phenol-formaldehyde (PF) Resins: While less common than UF resins, PF resins are sometimes used in particle board and MDF. They also emit formaldehyde, although at lower levels.

Isocyanates: Some particle boards and MDF products use polyurethane-based binders that contain isocyanates, which can cause respiratory problems and skin irritation.

Heavy Metals: Some adhesives and treatments used in particle board and MDF may contain heavy metals like lead, cadmium and mercury, which are toxic and can have severe health impacts.

Fire Retardants: Certain fire retardants used in these materials can contain toxic chemicals like polybrominated diphenyl ethers (PBDEs), which are linked to neurological and developmental issues.

Pesticides and Fungicides: Treated wood products, including particle board and MDF, may contain pesticides and fungicides to prevent insect and mould damage. These chemicals can off-gas and pose health risks.

Understanding these potential toxins is important for making informed decisions about the materials used in your baby's nursery, as prolonged exposure to these chemicals can negatively affect health, particularly for infants and young children.

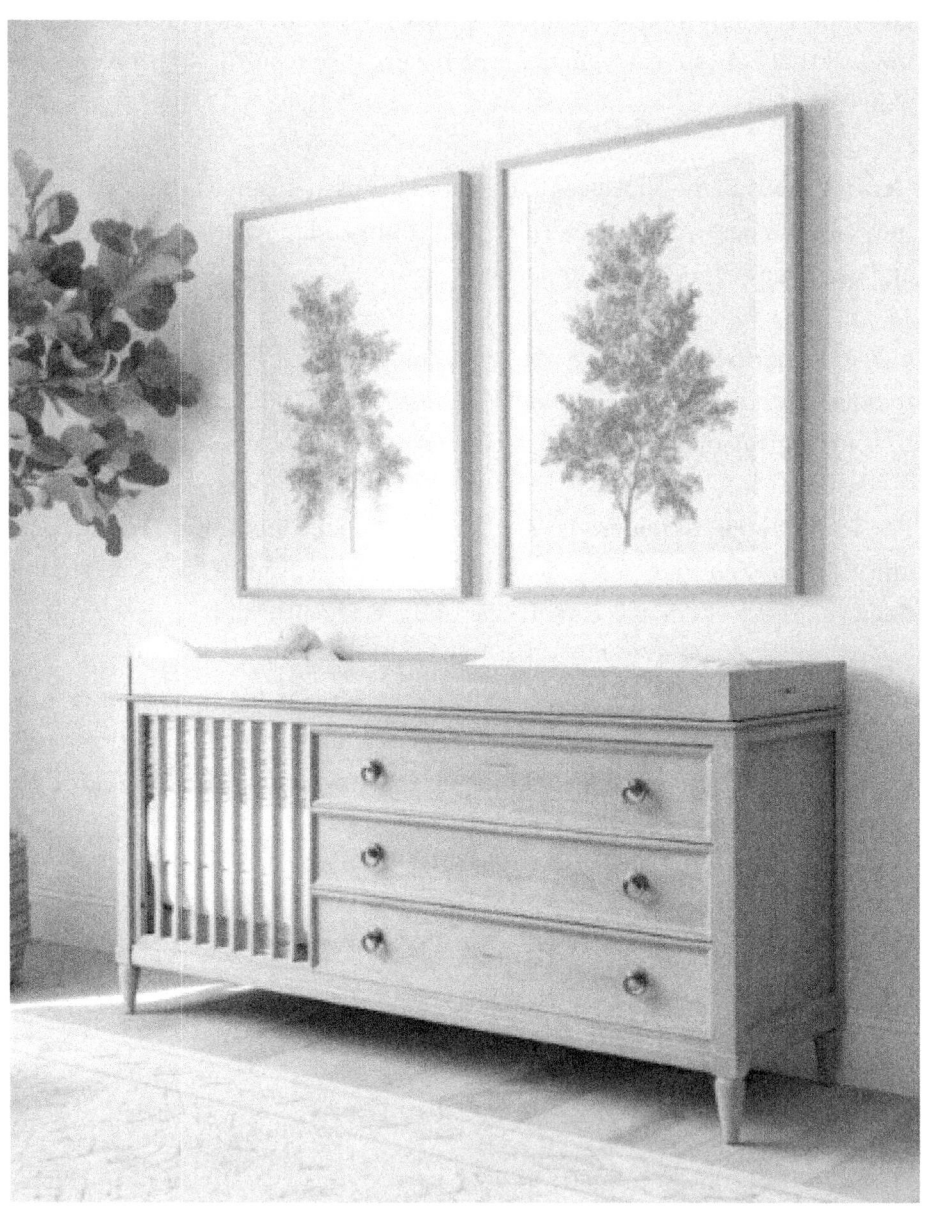

Non Toxic Paint and Wall Coverings

Using non toxic, low-VOC paint in a baby's nursery offers several important benefits. Low-VOC paints emit fewer volatile organic compounds, reducing indoor air pollution, minimising baby's exposure to harmful chemicals that can cause respiratory issues, allergies, headaches and other health problems. Babies have delicate skin, and reducing VOC exposure can help prevent skin irritations and allergic reactions.

Incorporating non-toxic, low-VOC paint in a baby's nursery is a proactive step toward ensuring a safe, healthy and comfortable environment for your child.

Low-VOC or Zero-VOC Paints
VOC (Volatile Organic Compounds) are chemicals that can off-gas and negatively impact indoor air quality. Look for paints labeled as low-VOC or zero-VOC.

Natural Paints
Natural paints are made from natural ingredients like plant oils, clay and chalk.

Natural Wallpaper
Choose wallpapers made from natural fibres and printed with water-based inks. Avoid all types of vinyl wallpaper as these can emit VOC's and other chemicals.

Eco Friendly Floor Coverings

Flooring
Consider natural flooring options such as hardwood, bamboo, or cork in the home, and particularly in baby's nursery. Ensure they are finished with non-toxic sealants.

Choose rugs or carpets made from natural fibres such as wool, cotton, or jute, making sure they are free from synthetic dyes and chemicals.

Cork Flooring

Cork is harvested from the bark of cork oak trees, which regrows, making it a renewable resource, that is naturally hypoallergenic and resistant to mould and mildew. Cork is soft underfoot and has natural cushioning, making it ideal for walking, standing and playtime.

Bamboo Flooring

Bamboo is a fast-growing grass, making it a highly renewable resource, and is harder and more durable than many hardwoods. If choosing bamboo flooring, ensure it has a low-VOC finish for indoor air quality.

Hardwood Flooring

When choosing hardwood flooring, opt for FSC-certified hardwood to ensure the wood is sourced from responsibly managed forests, and has non toxic finishes and sealants. Hardwood is long-lasting and can be refinished multiple times.

Linoleum

Sustainable linoleum is made from natural materials like linseed oil, wood flour, and cork dust. It is anti-bacterial and biodegradable, and very durable, lasting for decades with proper care.

Pure Wool Carpet

Wool is a natural, renewable fibre. It is soft and warm underfoot, providing a comfortable surface to walk on and for baby to play on. Pure wool is naturally flame-resistant and hypoallergenic.

Reclaimed Wood Flooring

Reclaimed wood adds a unique, rustic charm to baby's nursery. Reclaimed wood flooring reduces the demand for new lumber, thereby helping to preserve forests. Ensure the reclaimed wood is finished with non-toxic, low-VOC sealants for improved indoor air quality.

Rubber Flooring

Rubber flooring is often made from recycled rubber, such as old tyres. It is a soft and cushioned surface that is easy and safe for your baby to crawl and play on.

Non Toxic Adhesives and Finishes

When installing any type of flooring, use non toxic adhesives and finishes to ensure good indoor air quality. Ensure proper ventilation during and after installation to help dissipate any residual odours or chemicals.

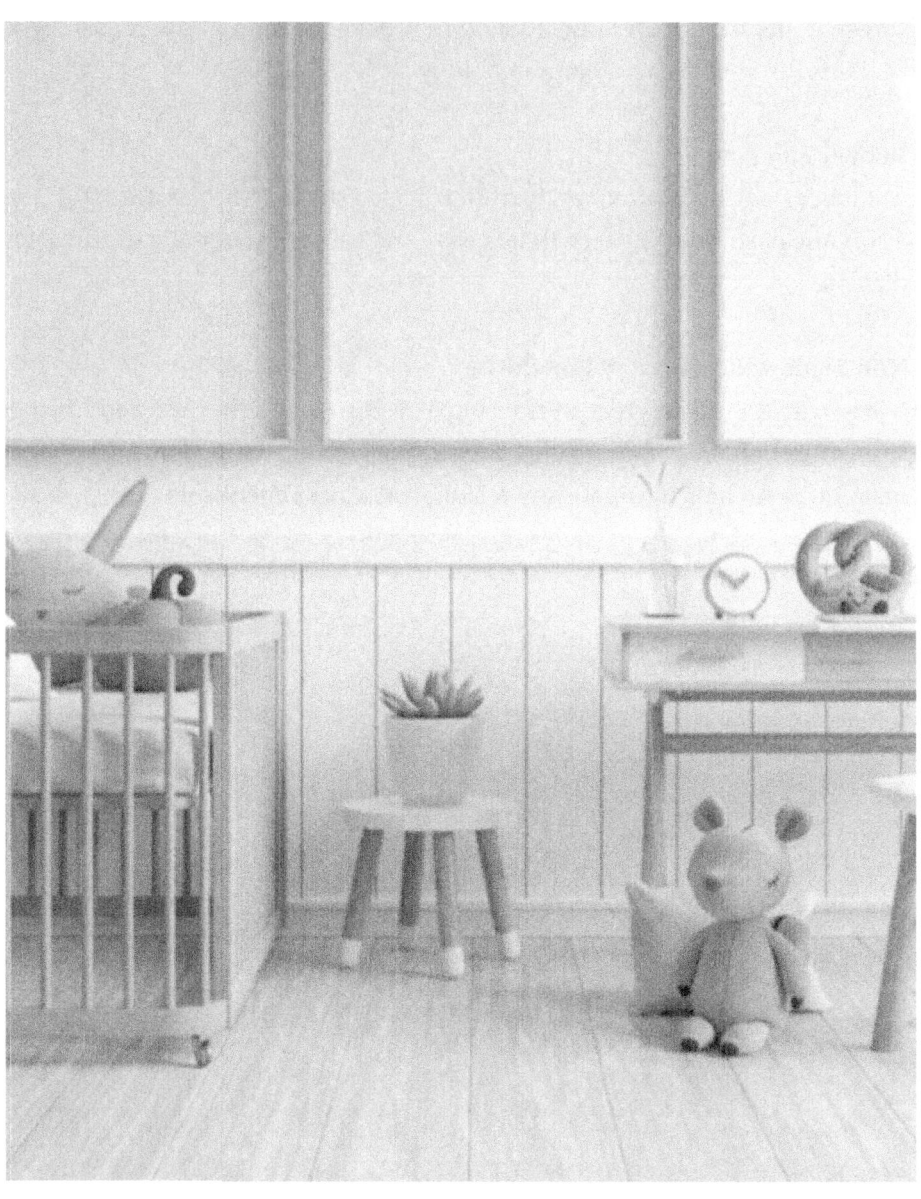

Natural & Non Toxic Bedding and Fabrics

Selecting non toxic and organic bedding and mattresses for your baby's nursery is an essential step in creating a safe and healthy sleep environment. These products are free from harmful chemicals and synthetic materials, reducing the risk of exposure to toxins that can affect your baby's health and development.

Organic bedding and mattresses are naturally hypoallergenic and breathable, offering superior comfort and reducing the likelihood of allergies and respiratory issues. Prioritising non toxic and organic bedding provides peace of mind, knowing your baby is resting and sleeping in a safe, nurturing space.

Bedding

Organic Cotton:
 Choose bedding and fabrics made from organic cotton. These are free from pesticides and harmful chemicals.

Natural Fibres:
 Consider materials like bamboo, hemp or wool.
Certifications:
 Look for certifications like GOTS (Global Organic Textile Standard) or OEKO-TEX Standard 100.

Mattresses:

Organic Cotton or Natural Latex:
 Choose mattresses made from organic cotton or natural latex. Ensure they are free from flame retardants and other harmful chemicals.
Certifications:
 Look for GREENGUARD Gold certification for low chemical emissions.

Benefits of Choosing Quality Bedding

- Non toxic and organic bedding and mattresses are free from harmful chemicals, reducing the risk of exposure to toxins that can affect your baby's health and development.
- Organic materials, such as cotton and wool, are naturally hypoallergenic and resistant to dust mites, mould, and mildew, which helps prevent allergies and respiratory issues.
- Organic bedding and mattresses allow for better air circulation, helping to regulate body temperature and keep baby comfortable throughout the night.
- Organic materials are often softer and more comfortable against your baby's sensitive skin, enhancing the quality of sleep and overall wellbeing.
- High-quality organic bedding and mattresses are often more durable, providing long-lasting comfort and support, which is both cost-effective and environmentally friendly.
- Organic products are made using sustainable farming practices that do not rely on harmful pesticides or synthetic fertilisers, promoting a healthier planet.
- As a parent you can rest assured knowing your baby is sleeping on safe, chemical-free materials, contributing to overall peace of mind and reduced stress.
- Opting for non toxic and organic bedding and mattresses is a valuable investment in your baby's health, comfort and environmental sustainability.

Creating a Peaceful Sleep Environment for Baby

Creating a peaceful and healthy sleep environment for your baby involves thoughtful consideration of both the physical space and the practices you implement.

Choose Sustainable Furniture

Select furniture made from sustainable materials such as FSC-certified wood or bamboo. Look for cribs, dressers, and changing tables with non toxic finishes and sturdy construction that will last through multiple children.

Opt for Natural Textiles

Use bedding, curtains and rugs made from organic cotton, bamboo or linen. These natural fibres are breathable, hypoallergenic and free from harmful chemicals, creating a cosy and comfortable sleep environment for your baby.

Maximise Natural Light

Position your baby's crib or bassinet near a window to take advantage of natural light during the day. Use sheer curtains or blinds to filter sunlight and create a soothing ambiance while allowing your baby to experience the natural rhythm of day and night.

Create a Calm Colour Palette

Choose soft, muted colours for the nursery walls and decor to promote relaxation and tranquility. Shades of blue, green, cream or lavender are calming and conducive to sleep. Avoid using overly stimulating or bright colours.

Use Eco Friendly Decor

Decorate the nursery with eco friendly decor such as handmade artwork, wooden toys and air purifying plants. Incorporate natural elements like woven baskets, rattan accents and live plants to bring a sense of nature indoors and create a peaceful atmosphere.

Invest in Energy-Efficient Lighting

Install energy-efficient LED light bulbs and use dimmer switches or night lights with adjustable brightness to create a gentle and soothing sleep environment. Avoid harsh overhead lighting and opt for soft, warm lighting in the evening to signal bedtime.

Minimise Electronic Devices

Keep electronic devices, such as TVs, computers and smartphones, out of the nursery to reduce exposure to blue light and electromagnetic radiation, which can disrupt sleep patterns. Create a screen-free zone to encourage relaxation and quality sleep.

Establish a Bedtime Routine

Develop a consistent bedtime routine that includes calming activities such as bath time, gentle massage and reading bedtime stories. Stick to a regular schedule to help regulate your baby's circadian rhythm and promote better sleep quality.

Encourage Natural Ventilation

Keep the nursery well-ventilated by opening windows or using a fan to promote air circulation and prevent overheating. Use breathable bedding and clothing to help regulate your baby's body temperature and create a comfortable sleep environment.

Sleep Routines for Eco Babies

Creating a sleep routine and implementing sustainable practices for eco-conscious babies involves integrating environmentally friendly choices into your baby's bedtime routine while prioritising their health and wellbeing.

Natural Bedtime Products: Use natural and organic baby products such as gentle bath wash, shampoo and baby lotion made from plant-based ingredients. Look for products that are free from toxic chemicals, synthetic fragrances and artificial dyes to nurture your baby's skin.

Toxin Free Bedtime Clothing: Dress your baby in organic cotton or bamboo sleepwear that is soft, breathable and gentle on their skin. Ideally choose pyjamas made from eco-sustainable materials and free from harmful chemicals to ensure a comfortable and safe sleep environment.

Reduce Electronic Exposure: Minimise exposure to electronic devices such as TVs, tablets, and smartphones before bedtime, as blue light can disrupt your baby's sleep-wake cycle. Instead, engage in screen-free activities such as reading books, listening to soft music or singing lullabies to encourage relaxation.

Create a Peaceful Sleep Environment: Set up a peaceful sleep environment by dimming the lights, playing soft music or white noise, and ensuring the room is cool, quiet and comfortable for sleep. Use blackout curtains or shades to block out light and create a dark, restful atmosphere for your baby.

Consistent Bedtime Routine: Establish a consistent bedtime routine that includes calming activities such as a warm bath, gentle massage or bedtime story to help your baby relax and unwind before sleep. Stick to a regular schedule to help regulate your baby's sleep-wake cycle and promote better sleep quality.

Encourage Self-Soothing: Allow your baby to learn self-soothing techniques such as sucking on a pacifier or thumb, cuddling with a favourite toy or blanket or gentle rocking to help them settle themselves to sleep. Avoid over-stimulation and excessive intervention to promote independent sleep skills.

Comfortable Sleep Surface: Choose a comfortable and supportive crib mattress made from natural and non toxic materials such as organic cotton, wool or natural latex. Ensure the crib is free from hazards such as loose bedding, stuffed animals or crib bumpers to reduce the risk of suffocation and promote safe sleep practices.

Monitor Room Temperature: Keep the nursery at a comfortable temperature between 68-72°F (20-22°C) to promote restful sleep. Use a room thermometer to monitor temperature levels and adjust bedding or clothing as needed to keep your baby comfortable throughout the night.

Practice Patience and Consistency: Be patient and consistent in implementing your baby's sleep routine, as it may take time for them to adjust and develop healthy sleep habits. Stay positive and supportive, and trust that with time and consistency, your baby will learn to settle themselves to sleep, and sleep through the night.

Eco-Friendly Sleep Products: Choose eco-friendly sleep products such as organic crib sheets, mattress protectors and sleep sacks made from sustainable materials. Look for certifications such as Global Organic Textile Standard (GOTS) to ensure that the products meet strict health and safety standards.

Co-Sleeping Safety

Co-sleeping and bed sharing can be a wonderful way to bond with your baby and promote breastfeeding, but it's important to prioritise safety to reduce the risk of accidents or suffocation.

Ensure a Firm Mattress: Use a firm mattress with a tight-fitting sheet in the adult bed to provide a safe sleeping surface for your baby. Avoid soft mattresses, waterbeds or sofas, as they can pose a suffocation hazard.

Create a Safe Sleep Environment: Keep pillows, blankets and other soft bedding away from your baby's sleeping area to reduce the risk of suffocation or entrapment. Use lightweight blankets or sleep sacks instead of heavy comforters.

Position Your Baby Safely: Place your baby on their back to sleep, with their head and face uncovered. Avoid placing your baby on their side or stomach, as this increases the risk of suffocation. Ensure that there are no gaps between the mattress and the bed frame or headboard where your baby could become trapped.

Stay Sober: Avoid co-sleeping or bed sharing if you have been drinking alcohol, using drugs or taking medications that could impair your judgement or coordination. Alcohol and drugs can interfere with your ability to respond to your baby's needs and increase the risk of accidental suffocation or injury.

Avoid Overheating: Dress your baby in lightweight, breathable sleepwear and keep the room at a comfortable temperature to prevent overheating. Avoid using heavy blankets or placing your baby near heaters or heating vents.

Keep Siblings and Pets Away: If you have other children or pets, ensure that they are not allowed to sleep in the same bed as your baby. Siblings and pets can accidentally roll onto or smother a sleeping baby.

Follow Safe Sleep Practices: Even when bed sharing or co- sleeping, it's important to follow safe sleep practices recommended by pediatricians, such as placing your baby on a firm, flat surface with no soft bedding or pillows.

Trust Your Instincts: If you feel uncomfortable or unsure about co-sleeping or bed sharing, trust your instincts and consider alternative sleeping arrangements such as a bassinet or co-sleeper attached to the side of the adult bed. It's important to prioritise safety and choose the sleeping arrangement that works best for your family.

By following these safety guidelines, you can reduce the risk of accidents or suffocation while co-sleeping or bed sharing with your baby, allowing you to enjoy the benefits of close, nurturing sleep while keeping your little one safe and protected.

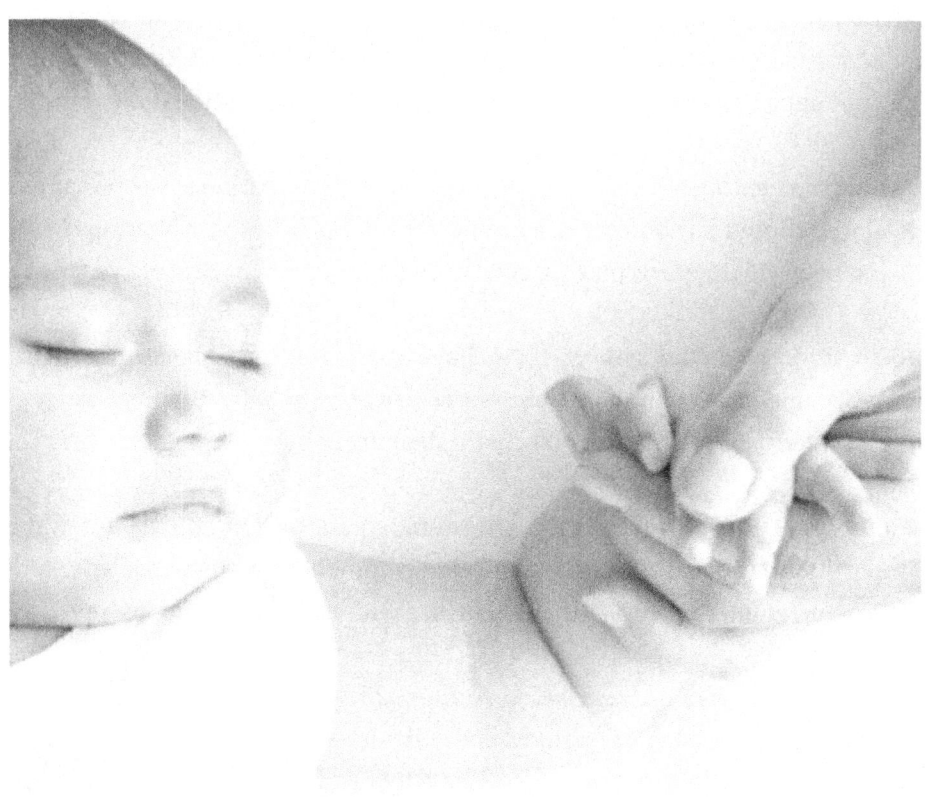

Maximising Natural Light & Energy Efficiency

Maximising natural light in your baby's nursery not only creates a bright and cheerful atmosphere but also has numerous benefits for your baby's health and wellbeing.

Choose the Right Window Treatments

Opt for sheer curtains or blinds that allow natural light to filter through while still providing privacy. Consider light-coloured or translucent window coverings that reflect light into the room. Install adjustable blinds or shades that can be easily opened during the day to let in sunlight and closed at night for privacy.

Keep Windows Clean and Unobstructed

Regularly clean windows to remove dirt and grime that can obstruct sunlight. Avoid placing furniture or bulky items in front of windows to allow maximum light penetration into the room.

Use Mirrors to Reflect Light

Position mirrors strategically to reflect natural light into darker areas of the room. Choose large, decorative mirrors to enhance the sense of brightness and spaciousness in the nursery.

Paint Walls in Light Colours

Choose light-colored paint for walls, such as white, pastel shades or soft neutrals, to maximise light reflection. Consider using non-toxic or low-VOC paint with a satin or glossy finish, which reflects more light compared to matte finishes.

Ventilation

Ensure proper ventilation in the nursery to reduce any potential off-gassing from new materials.

Minimise Obstructions

Keep furniture, decor and accessories to a minimum to avoid blocking natural light flow. Choose low-profile furniture and open shelving to maintain an open and airy feel in the nursery.

Utilise Skylights or Sun Tunnels

Install skylights or sun tunnels to bring additional natural light into the nursery from above. Consider energy-efficient options with built-in blinds or shades for control over light levels and privacy.

Trim Trees and Bushes Outside Windows

Trim overhanging branches and bushes outside windows to allow more sunlight to enter the room. Consider planting light-coloured or reflective foliage to enhance natural light reflection.

Create Light-Enhancing Decor

Choose light-coloured flooring, such as hardwood or light-coloured, natural-fibre carpet, to reflect natural light. Decorate with shiny or metallic accents to bounce light around the room and create a sparkling effect.

Install Translucent Doors or Room Dividers

Use translucent doors or room dividers to allow natural light to flow freely between spaces while still providing privacy. Consider options like glass-panelled doors or sliding doors with frosted glass inserts.

Incorporate Natural Elements

Decorate with natural materials like wood, bamboo and rattan to enhance the connection to the outdoors and complement natural light. Place potted plants strategically near windows to filter light and improve indoor air quality.

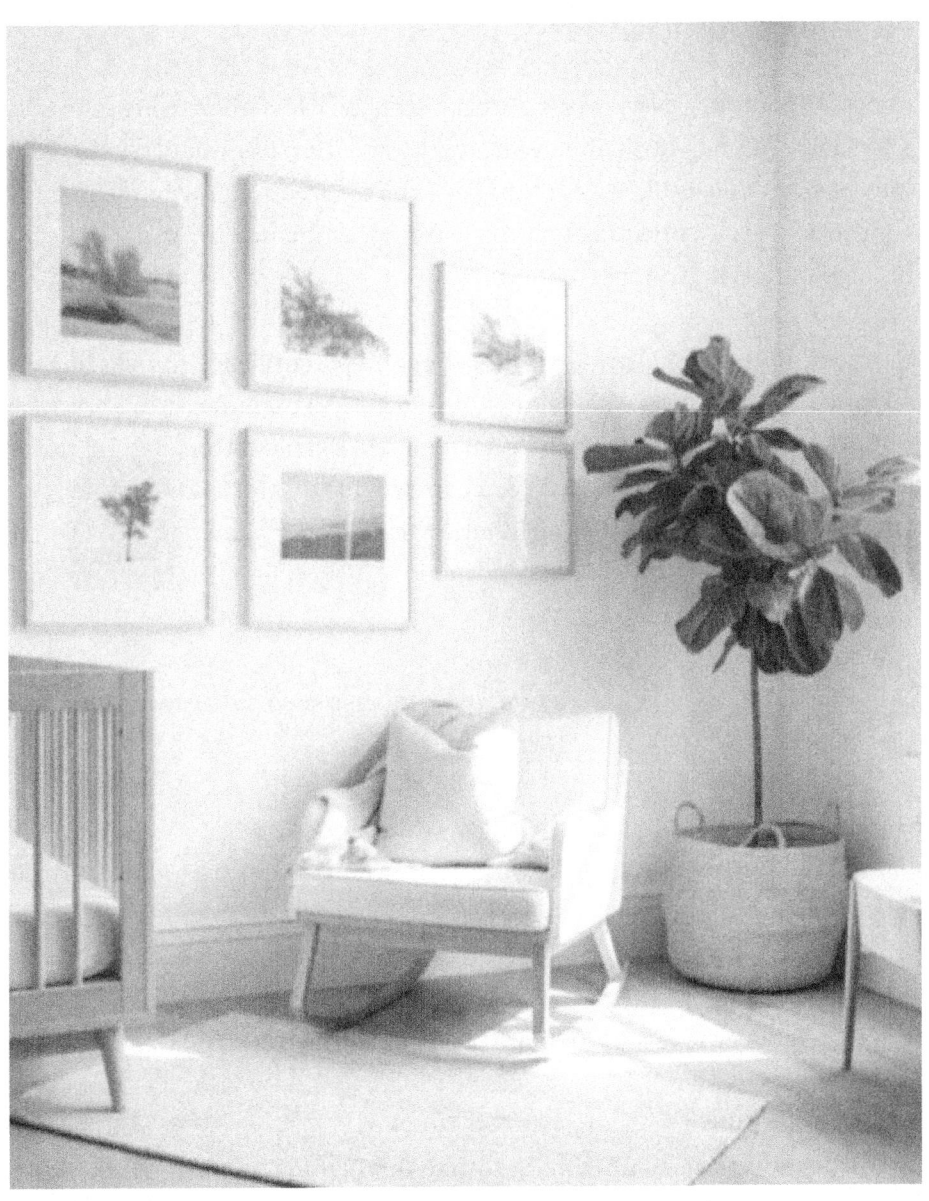

Non Toxic Toys for Baby

Choosing non-toxic baby toys is a crucial decision when prioritising the health and safety of your little one. With the growing awareness of the harmful effects of chemicals like BPA, phthalates and lead, commonly found in many conventional toys, selecting toys made from natural, non toxic materials has become increasingly important.

Non toxic toys not only protect your baby from potential health risks but also supports environmental sustainability and ethical manufacturing practices. By opting for toys made from materials such as organic cotton, natural rubber and sustainably sourced wood, you can provide a safer and healthier play environment for baby while contributing to a greener planet.

Choose toys made from:

Wood:
Opt for solid wood toys with non toxic finishes such as beeswax or natural oils.

Organic Cotton:
Toys made from 100% organic cotton are safe and free from harmful chemicals.

Natural Rubber:
Natural rubber toys are free from plasticisers and other toxic chemicals.

Food-Grade Silicone:
Silicone toys, especially those that are food-grade, are safe for babies to chew on.

Stainless Steel:
For items like rattles or utensils, stainless steel is a safe and durable option.

Non Toxic Toys for Baby's Health and Safety

Reduced Exposure to Harmful Chemicals:
Non toxic toys are free from harmful substances such as BPA, phthalates, lead and PVC, reducing the risk of exposure to these chemicals.

Safe for Chewing:
Babies often explore toys with their mouths. Non toxic toys made from materials like organic cotton, natural rubber and food-grade silicone are safe for chewing and teething.

Lower Allergy Risk:
Non toxic toys, particularly those made from natural materials, are less likely to contain allergens that could trigger reactions in sensitive children.

Stimulating Play:
Non toxic toys often have textures and forms that enhance sensory development and fine motor skills.

Encourages Imaginative Play:
Simple toys, like wooden blocks and cloth dolls, encourage imaginative and open-ended play, fostering creativity and problem-solving skills.

Long-Lasting:
Toys made from high-quality materials, such as solid wood and organic fabrics, are generally more durable and can withstand rough play, leading to longer use.

Heirloom Potential:
High-quality, non toxic toys can be passed down through generations, providing lasting value and reducing the need for frequent replacements.

DIY Eco Friendly Baby Toys

Making your own eco-friendly toys for your baby is a wonderful way to provide them with healthy and sustainable playthings while minimising environmental impact.

Fabric Sensory Balls:
Materials

Organic cotton fabric scraps

Sewing machine or needle and thread Scissors

Filling material (organic cotton batting or wool)

Instructions

Cut fabric scraps into squares or circles of equal size. Place two fabric pieces together with the right sides facing each other.

Sew around the edges, leaving a small opening.

Turn the fabric inside out through the opening.

Fill the fabric ball with stuffing material.

Hand stitch the opening closed.

Wooden Teething Ring:
Materials

Untreated wooden ring (such as a wooden curtain ring) Organic cotton fabric strip

Organic beeswax or coconut oil (optional)

Instructions

Wrap the wooden ring tightly with the fabric strip, covering the entire surface.

Tie the ends of the fabric strip in a knot to secure.

Optionally, apply a thin layer of organic beeswax or coconut oil to the fabric to protect it and make it more resistant to drool.

Crochet Bunny Rabbit
Materials

Worsted weight yarn in desired colour (organic cotton or wool yarn recommended)

Crochet hook appropriate for your yarn weight (size H/5.00mm recommended)

Fibrefill stuffing (organic cotton batting or wool recommended)

Yarn needle

Scissors

Body of Bunny Rabbit:

Begin with a magic ring.

Round 1:

Work 6 single crochet (sc) stitches into the magic ring. (6 stitches)

Round 2:

Work 2 sc into each stitch around. (12 stitches)

Rounds 3-6:

Work 1 sc into each stitch around. (12 stitches)

Round 7:

Work 1 sc into the next stitch, then 2 sc into the next stitch. Repeat from * to * around. (18 stitches)

Rounds 8-12:

Work 1 sc into each stitch around. (18 stitches)

Round 13:

Work 1 sc into each of the next 2 stitches, then 2 sc into the next stitch. Repeat from * to * around. (24 stitches)

Rounds 14-17:

Work 1 sc into each stitch around. (24 stitches)

Round 18:

Work 1 sc into each of the next 2 stitches, then sc2tog (single crochet two stitches together) over the next 2 stitches. Repeat from * to * around. (18 stitches)

Stuff the body firmly with fibrefill stuffing.

Round 19:

Work 1 sc into the next stitch, then sc2tog over the next 2 stitches. Repeat from * to * around. (12 stitches)

Round 20:

Sc2tog over the next 2 stitches. Repeat from * to * around. (6 stitches)

Fasten off, leaving a long tail. Use the tail to close the opening by weaving it through the remaining stitches and pulling tight. Secure and weave in ends.

Ears (make 2):

Begin with a magic ring.

Round 1:

Work 6 single crochet (sc) stitches into the magic ring. (6 stitches)

Round 2:

Work 2 sc into each stitch around. (12 stitches)

Round 3:

Work 1 sc into the next stitch, then 2 sc into the next stitch. Repeat from * to * around. (18 stitches)

Rounds 4-5:

Work 1 sc into each stitch around. (18 stitches)

Fasten off, leaving a long tail for sewing. Flatten the ears and sew them onto the top of the bunny's head.

Face:

Use black yarn to embroider eyes and a nose onto the bunny's face. You can also add a mouth if desired.

Your crochet bunny rabbit stuffed animal is now complete! Adjust the size of the finished toy by using thicker or thinner yarn and a corresponding hook size. Always ensure that all parts are securely attached and avoid using small parts or buttons that could pose a choking hazard for young children.

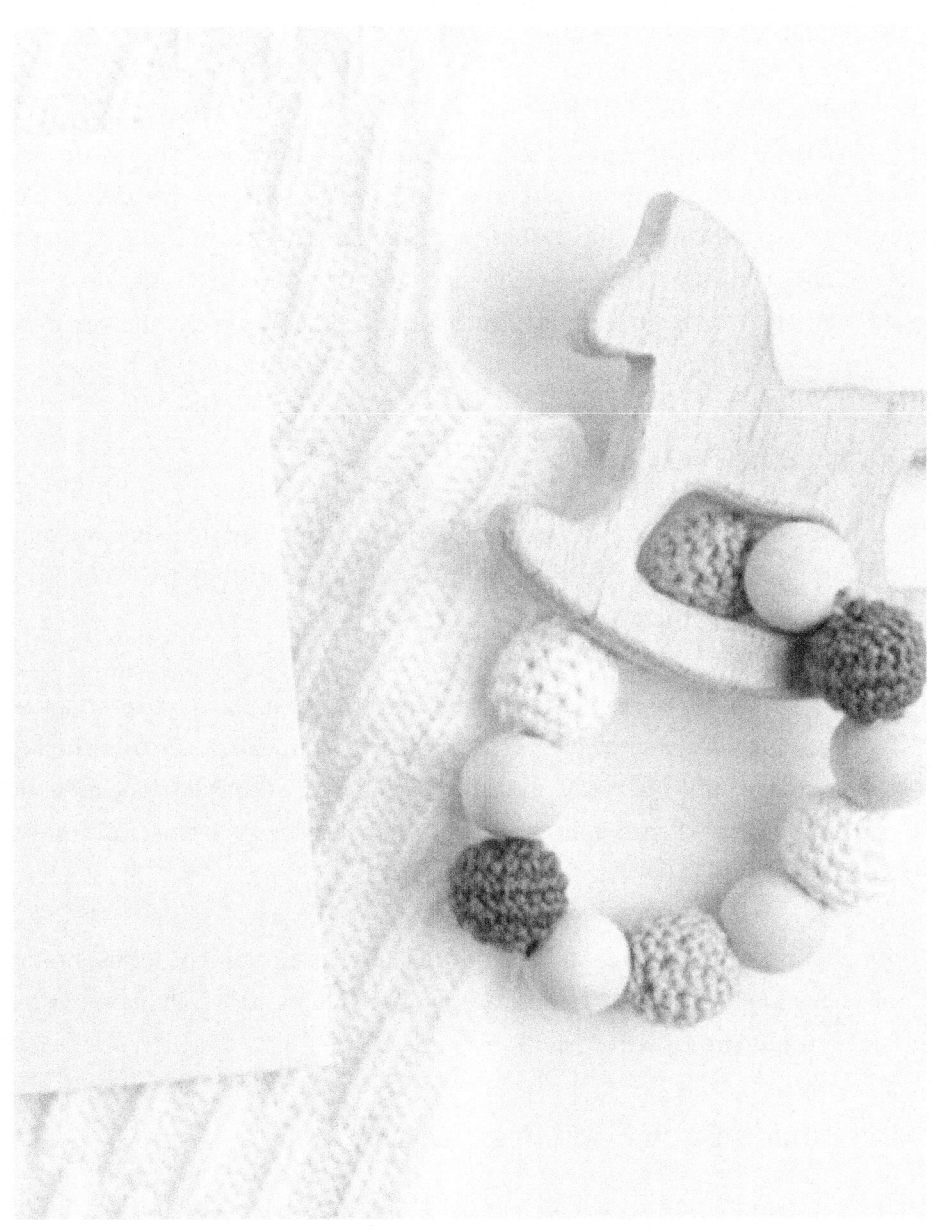

Nourishing Your Eco Baby

Welcoming a new addition to the family is a joyous occasion, accompanied by a myriad of decisions aimed at ensuring the wellbeing of your little one. As a toxin free eco-parent, nurturing your baby extends beyond love and physical care; it includes a nourishing environment that prioritises long-term health and environmental consciousness. Every choice, from the food you feed your baby, to the products you select, to the practices you embrace, holds the potential to shape a happier, more vibrant future for your child.

Organic Baby Food

Embarking on the adventure of introducing your baby to solid foods is not only a milestone in their development but also an opportunity to instill healthy eating habits from the start.

Choosing organic and homemade baby food offers a plethora of benefits, ensuring your little one receives nutritionally-rich meals while minimising exposure to harmful chemicals and additives. By preparing baby food at home using organic ingredients, sourced locally when possible, you have full control over the quality and freshness of each meal.

From vibrant fruits and vegetables to wholesome grains and proteins, homemade baby food allows you to tailor recipes to suit your baby's evolving tastes and nutritional needs.

Homemade Baby Food Recipes

Here are eight recipes for homemade organic baby food, covering a range of flavours and nutrients suitable for various stages of your baby's development:

Avocado Banana Mash
  1 ripe organic avocado

1 ripe organic banana

Mash the avocado and banana together until smooth. Serve immediately or store in an airtight container in the refrigerator for up to 24 hours.

Sweet Potato Puree

1 medium organic sweet potato

Peel and chop the sweet potato into small cubes. Steam until tender, then puree in a blender or food processor until smooth. Add a little filtered water or breast milk to achieve the desired consistency.

Apple Pear Sauce

1 organic apple

1 organic pear

Peel, core and chop the apple and pear. Steam until soft, then puree until smooth.

Carrot and Broccoli Mash

1 organic carrot

1 cup organic broccoli florets

Peel and chop the carrot, then steam with the broccoli until both are tender. Blend together until smooth, adding filtered water or breast milk as needed.

Quinoa and Banana Porridge

2 tablespoons organic quinoa

1 ripe organic banana

1/2 cup filtered water or breast milk

Rinse the quinoa thoroughly. Cook in water or breast milk until tender. Mash the banana and stir into the cooked quinoa until well combined.

Spinach and Pea Puree

1 cup organic spinach leaves

1/2 cup organic peas (fresh or frozen)

Steam the spinach and peas until tender. Blend together until smooth, adding filtered water or breast milk as needed to reach the desired consistency.

Blueberry Oatmeal

    2 tablespoons organic rolled oats
    1/4 cup filtered water or breast milk
    1/4 cup organic blueberries

Cook the oats in water or breast milk until soft. Mash the blueberries and stir into the cooked oatmeal.

Pumpkin and Banana Mash

    1/2 cup organic pumpkin puree
    1 ripe organic banana

Mix the pumpkin puree with mashed banana until smooth. Serve immediately or store in an airtight container in the refrigerator for up to 24 hours.

These homemade organic baby food recipes provide a nutritious and delicious start for your little one's culinary journey, ensuring they receive the best possible start to a lifetime of healthy eating.

Sustainable & Non Toxic Feeding Accessories

Choosing sustainable and non toxic feeding accessories for your baby is a wonderful way to ensure the health and safety of your little one, while reducing your environmental footprint.

Bamboo or Silicone Bibs

Use bibs made from organic cotton, bamboo or silicone, as these materials are safer and more sustainable than traditional plastics. Look for bibs that are easy to clean and durable for long-term use.

Glass Baby Bottles

Instead of plastic bottles, consider using glass baby bottles, which are free from harmful chemicals like BPA and phthalates. Glass is also recyclable and more eco-friendly than plastic.

Stainless Steel or Silicone Feeding Spoons

Choose feeding spoons made from stainless steel or silicone, as these materials are non toxic and durable. Avoid plastic spoons, which can leach harmful chemicals into your baby's food and into their body.

Reusable Food Pouches

Instead of single-use disposable pouches, opt for reusable food pouches made from food-grade silicone. These pouches are reusable, refillable, dishwasher-safe and reduce waste and plastic pollution.

Organic Cotton Burp Cloths

Choose burp cloths made from organic cotton, as conventional cotton production can be harmful to the environment due to pesticide use. Organic cotton is grown without synthetic pesticides or fertilisers, making it healthier for baby and a more sustainable choice.

Wooden High Chairs

Consider investing in a wooden high chair made from sustainably sourced wood instead of toxin-harbouring plastic. Wooden high chairs are durable, long-lasting and biodegradable at the end of their lifespan.

Silicone Sippy Cups

Look for sippy cups made from food-grade silicone, as silicone is durable, non toxic and easy to clean. Avoid sippy cups with plastic valves or straws, which can harbour bacteria and may contain harmful chemicals.

Natural Rubber Pacifiers

Choose pacifiers made from natural rubber instead of synthetic materials like plastic. Natural rubber is biodegradable and derived from sustainable sources like the rubber tree.

Cloth Nursing Pads

If you're breastfeeding, opt for cloth nursing pads made from organic cotton or bamboo instead of disposable pads. Cloth nursing pads are reusable, washable and reduce waste.

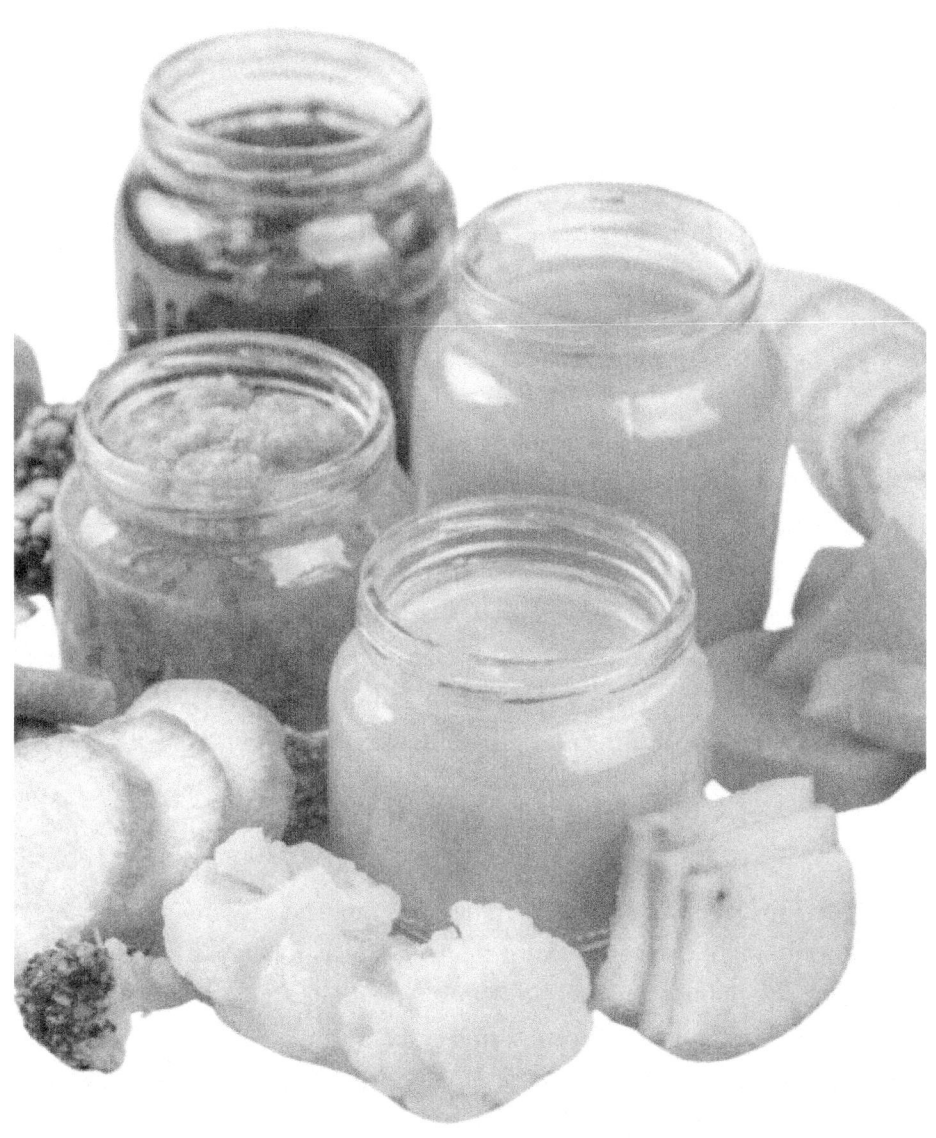

Cloth vs. Disposable Diapers (Nappies)

The choice between cloth diapers and disposable diapers is often a personal one, influenced by factors such as convenience, cost, environmental impact and personal preferences.

Cloth Diapers (Nappies)

Cloth diapers are often considered more environmentally friendly because they can be reused multiple times, reducing the amount of waste sent to landfills. While cloth diapers have a higher upfront cost, they can save money in the long run, especially if they are used for multiple children.

Cloth diapers are typically made from natural, breathable materials like cotton or bamboo, which may be gentler on baby's skin and less likely to cause irritation or allergic reactions. Consider that cloth diapers require regular washing, which can be time-consuming and may increase water and energy usage. However, modern cloth diapering systems have become more convenient with the availability of diaper liners and diaper services. Cloth diapers now come in a variety of styles, including prefolds, fitted, pocket and all-in-one diapers, allowing parents to choose the option that best suits their baby's needs and their lifestyle.

Disposable Diapers (Nappies)

Disposable diapers are convenient because they are easy to use and require no additional laundering or maintenance. This can be particularly helpful for parents with busy lifestyles or those who do not have access to laundry facilities. There is the environmental impact to consider with disposable diapers, however, as they contribute to landfill waste and their production requires the use of non-renewable resources like petroleum. Consider purchasing disposable diaper brands that offer more eco friendly options, such as biodegradable materials or reduced packaging.

While disposable diapers have a lower upfront cost compared to cloth diapers, they can become a significant ongoing expense, especially for families with multiple children. Disposable diapers often contain chemicals like dyes, fragrances and absorbent gels, which may irritate sensitive skin or cause allergic reactions in some babies.

Disposable diapers typically have higher absorbency compared to cloth diapers, which can be beneficial for overnight use or for babies who urinate frequently.

Some families may choose to use a combination of both options, such as cloth diapers at home and disposable diapers while traveling or during nighttime.

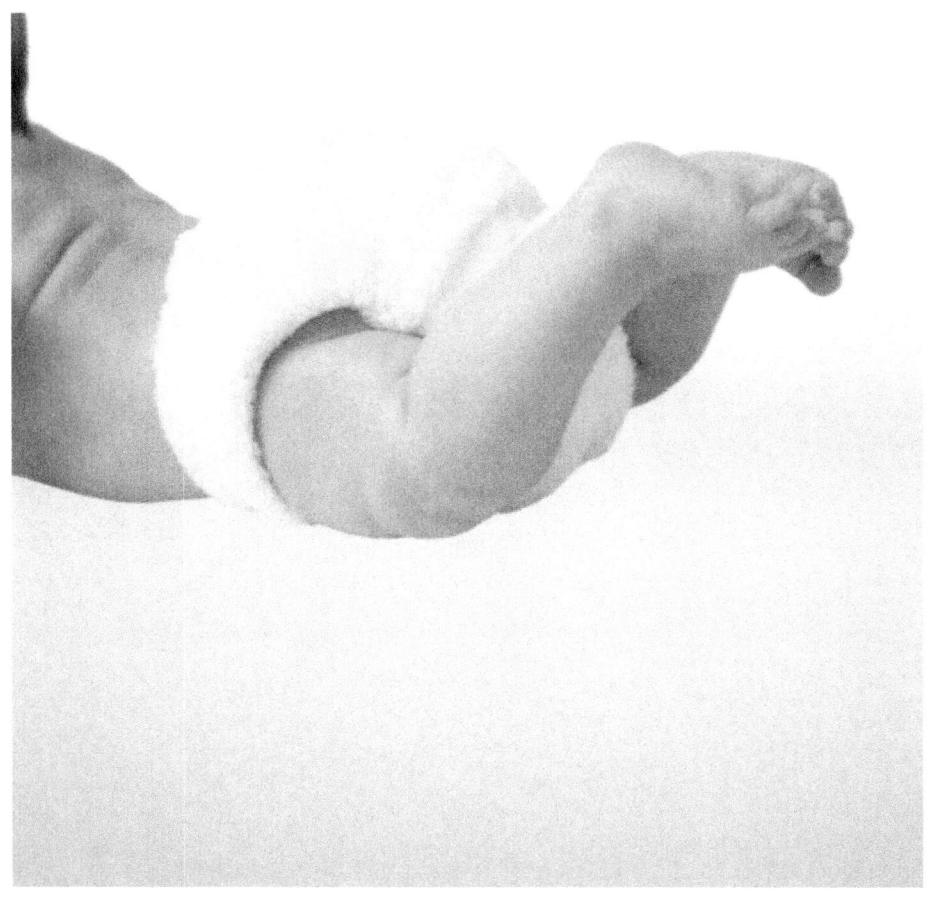

Non Toxic Bottle & Breastfeeding Practices

Practicing toxin free bottle feeding and breastfeeding involves making choices that prioritise the health and wellbeing of your baby.

Toxin Free and Eco Bottle Feeding

Choose bottles made from materials that are safe for your baby. Look for options made from glass or stainless steel, as these materials are free from harmful chemicals such as BPA and phthalates, are durable and recyclable.

Select bottle teats made from natural materials like silicone or rubber, which are free from harmful chemicals and are biodegradable at the end of their lifespan.

Minimise single-use waste by avoiding disposable bottle liners and single-serving formula packets. Instead, choose reusable bottle accessories such as silicone bottle sleeves or formula dispensers.

When sterilising bottles and accessories, opt for eco- friendly sterilisation methods such as boiling water or using steam sterilisers that consume less energy than traditional methods.

Consider donating gently used bottles and accessories to others in need, or re-purpose them for crafts or storage to extend their lifespan and avoid burdening landfills.

Breastfeeding

Breastfeeding inherently produces less waste compared to bottle feeding, as breast milk is produced and delivered in a sustainable, zero-waste manner.

Choose breastfeeding accessories made from natural materials, such as organic cotton nursing pads or reusable silicone breast milk storage bags, to minimise single-use waste.

If pumping breast milk, opt for a high-quality, durable breast pump that can be used for multiple children or shared with others to reduce the need for additional accessories.

Store expressed breast milk in glass or BPA-free plastic storage containers instead of disposable plastic bags to minimise waste and to reduce your baby's exposure to harmful chemicals.

Advocate for policies and initiatives that support breastfeeding-friendly environments in workplaces, public spaces and communities to promote breastfeeding as a sustainable feeding option.

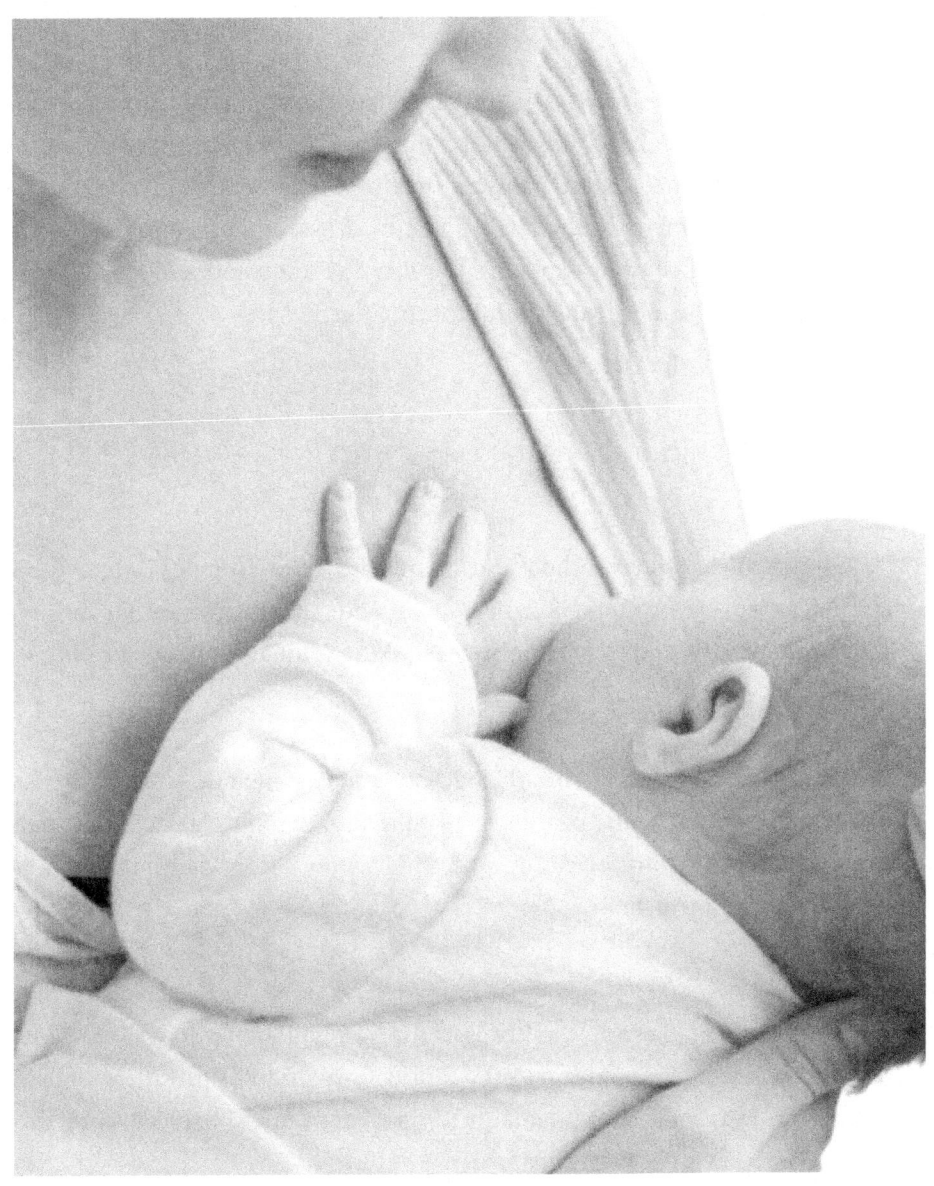

Dressing Your Eco Baby

With a growing awareness of the impact of synthetic 'fast fashion' on the environment, more parents are seeking non toxic clothing alternatives that prioritise the health of their baby and the planet. From organic fabrics to ethically made garments, every choice in dressing your baby offers an opportunity to reduce their exposure to synthetic, petroleum-based fabrics, and to support conscious, fair-trade clothing businesses.

Choosing Organic and Natural Fabrics

Organic Cotton:
Organic cotton is grown without the use of synthetic pesticides or fertilisers, making it safer for your baby's delicate skin and better for the environment. It's soft, breathable and easy to care for, making it ideal for baby clothing.

Bamboo:
Bamboo fabric is derived from the bamboo plant, which grows quickly and requires minimal water and pesticides to cultivate. Bamboo fabric is naturally hypoallergenic, moisture-wicking, and is incredibly soft, making it a popular choice for baby clothing.

Hemp:
Hemp fabric is made from the fibres of the hemp plant, which is known for its durability and sustainability. Hemp fabric is breathable, antimicrobial and becomes softer with each wash, making it a great option for baby clothing that can withstand frequent washing.

Organic Wool:
Organic wool is sourced from sheep raised on organic farms that avoid the use of synthetic chemicals, and adhere to strict animal welfare standards. Wool is naturally moisture-wicking, temperature-regulating and flame-resistant,

making it an excellent choice for baby clothing, especially in colder climates.

Tencel (Lyocell):
Tencel, also known as Lyocell, is a sustainable fabric made from wood pulp, typically sourced from eucalyptus or other fast-growing trees. Tencel is soft, breathable and biodegradable, making it a great eco friendly option for baby clothing.

Organic Linen:
Organic linen is made from the fibres of the flax plant and is known for its strength, breathability and moisture-wicking properties. Linen becomes softer and more comfortable with each wash, making it a great choice for baby clothing, especially in warmer climates.

When choosing organic and natural fabrics for your baby's clothing, look for certifications such as GOTS (Global Organic Textile Standard) or OEKO-TEX Standard 100, which ensure that the fabrics are free from harmful chemicals and produced in an environmentally and socially responsible manner.

Second Hand & Hand-Me-Down Clothing

Opting for second hand and hand-me-down options is a fantastic way to practice sustainability and reduce waste when dressing your eco baby.

Consignment Shops and Thrift Stores:
Visit local consignment shops and thrift stores to browse their selection of baby clothing. You can often find high-quality items at affordable prices, and shopping second-hand helps keep clothing out of landfills.

Online Marketplaces:
Explore online marketplaces like eBay, Facebook Marketplace, or Craigslist for pre-loved baby clothing. Many parents sell or give away gently used items that their children have outgrown, making it easy to find bargains from the

comfort of your home.

Clothing Swaps:

Organise or participate in clothing swaps with friends, family or other parents in your community. This allows you to exchange baby clothing that your child has outgrown for items that are new to you, all without spending a dime.

Hand-Me-Downs:

Accept hand-me-downs graciously from friends, family members or neighbors who have children slightly older than yours. Not only does this save money, but it also creates a sense of community and connection as you share in the joy of watching children grow.

Online Resale Platforms:

Explore online resale platforms specialising in children's clothing, such as Jumping Jack, ThredUp or Poshmark. These platforms offer a wide selection of gently used baby clothing from various brands and allow you to filter by size, style and condition.

Local Parenting Groups:

Join local parenting groups or online communities where parents buy, sell or trade baby clothing. These groups often have dedicated sections or threads for baby clothing, making it easy to connect with other parents in your area.

Family Heirlooms:

Consider using family heirlooms or sentimental clothing passed down from previous generations. These pieces may hold special meaning and add a unique touch to your baby's wardrobe while reducing the need for new purchases.

DIY Baby Clothing and Accessories

Creating your own DIY baby clothing and accessories is a fun and sustainable way to dress your little one, while reducing waste and embracing creativity.

Upcycled Clothing:
Give new life to old clothing by upcycling them into adorable baby outfits. For example, you can turn a worn-out adult sweater into a cozy baby cardigan or transform an old t-shirt into a cute baby romper.

Organic Fabric Projects:
Choose organic fabrics like cotton, bamboo or hemp to make homemade baby clothing and accessories. Sew simple garments like onesies, pants, or bibs using organic fabric and natural dyes for decoration.

Handmade Toys:
Create eco-friendly toys for your baby using natural materials like organic cotton, wool or wood. Sew soft toys, knit stuffed animals or make sensory toys using fabric scraps and non-toxic fillings.

DIY Baby Wraps and Slings:
Make your own baby wraps or slings using organic fabric. There are many tutorials available online that show you how to sew a simple wrap or sling that provides comfort and support for both you and your baby.

Homemade Hats and Booties:
Knit or crochet hats, booties and mittens for your baby using organic yarn. These handmade accessories are not only cute but also keep your baby warm and cosy during colder months.

Reusable Diaper Covers:
Sew reusable diaper covers using waterproof fabric like PUL (polyurethane laminate) or wool.

Natural Dyeing:

Experiment with natural dyeing techniques to colour organic fabrics for baby clothing and accessories. Use ingredients like avocado pits, onion skins, beetroot juice or turmeric to create beautiful, non toxic dyes that are safe for your baby's delicate skin.

Embroidery and Applique:

Add personalised touches to baby clothing and accessories through embroidery or applique. Embroider cute designs or your baby's name onto onesies, blankets or burp cloths, or applique fabric shapes onto clothing for a unique look.

DIY Baby Shower Gifts:

Create homemade baby clothing and accessories as thoughtful gifts for expecting friends or family members. Handmade gifts add a personal touch and show that you care about the wellbeing of both the baby and the planet.

By embracing DIY projects, you can create unique and sustainable clothing and accessories for your eco baby while fostering creativity and reducing your environmental impact. Search YouTube for tutorials on 'upcycling baby clothing'. There are many videos and tutorials available.

DIY Crochet Baby Hat

Materials

Worsted weight yarn in desired colour (organic cotton or wool yarn recommended)

Crochet hook appropriate for your yarn weight (size H/5.00mm recommended)

Yarn needle Scissors

Instructions

Note: This pattern is for a basic beanie-style baby hat, suitable for newborns to 6 months old. Adjustments can be made for larger sizes by increasing the number of stitches and/or rows.

Round 1:

Start with a magic ring. Chain 2 (counts as first half double crochet), then work 9 half double crochet (hdc) stitches into the magic ring.

Pull the ring closed. (10 stitches total)

Round 2:

Chain 2 (counts as first hdc), then work 1 hdc into the same stitch. Work 2 hdc into each stitch around.

Join with a slip stitch to the top of the beginning chain 2. (20 stitches total)

Round 3:

Chain 2 (counts as first hdc), then work 1 hdc into the same stitch. *Work 1 hdc into the next stitch, then 2 hdc into the following stitch.*

Repeat from * to * around. Join with a slip stitch to the top of the beginning chain 2. (30 stitches total)

Round 4-8:

Chain 2 (counts as first hdc), then work 1 hdc into each stitch around.

Join with a slip stitch to the top of the beginning chain 2. (30 stitches total for each round)

Round 9 (Optional):

To add a decorative edge, you can work a round of single crochet (sc) stitches around the bottom edge of the hat. Simply chain 1, then work 1 sc into each stitch around. Join with a slip stitch to the first sc. Fasten off and weave in ends.

Finishing: Fasten off, leaving a long tail for sewing. Thread the yarn tail onto a yarn needle and weave it through the stitches of the last round. Pull tight to close the top of the hat. Secure the yarn and weave in any remaining ends.

Optional Embellishments:

Add a pom-pom to the top of the hat for a fun and playful touch.

Attach a small crochet applique, such as a flower, to the side of the hat for decoration.

Crochet a contrasting colour edging around the bottom edge of the hat.

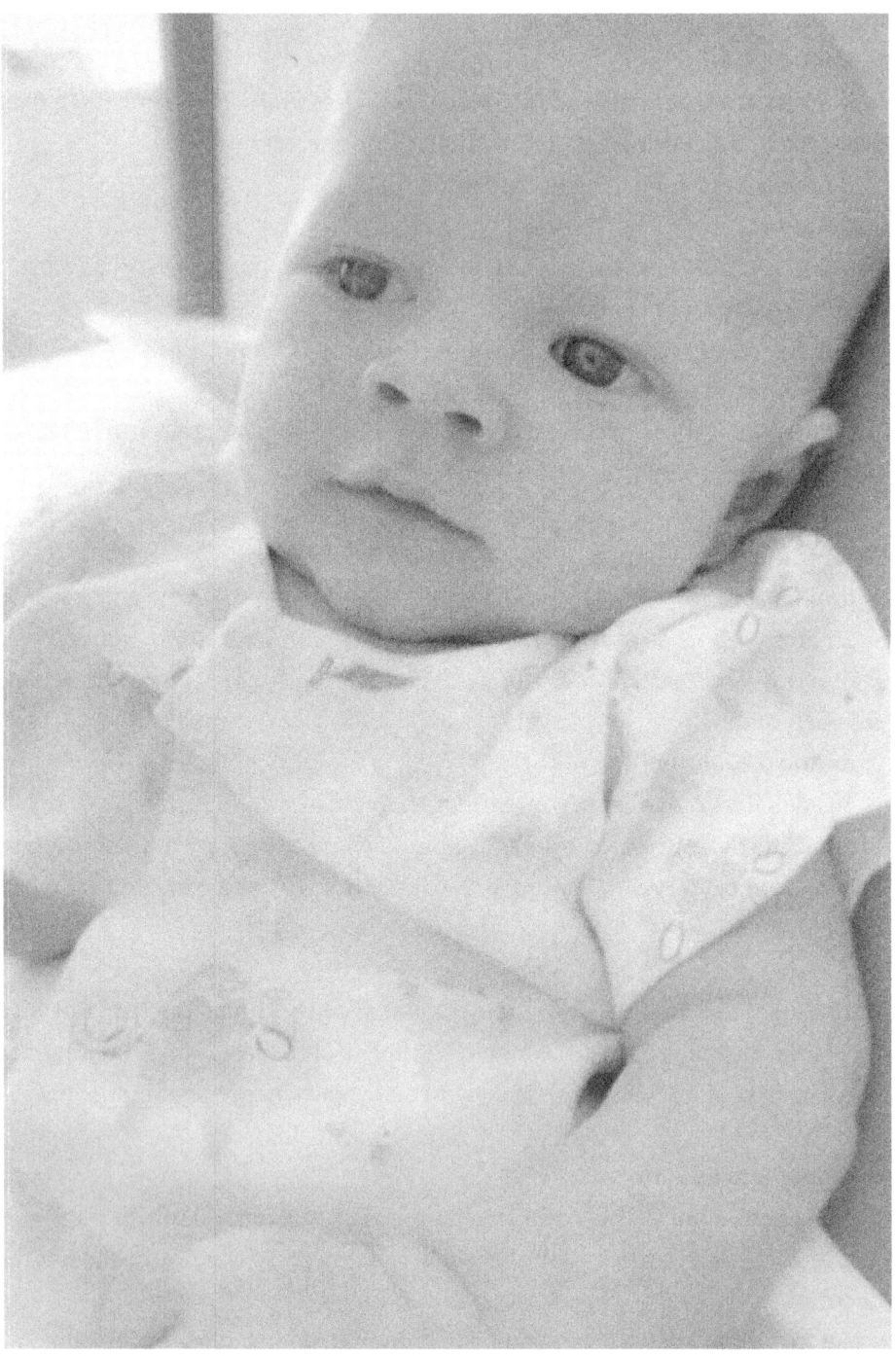

Eco-Friendly Baby Care

From the products you use to the practices you embrace, every aspect of caring for your baby can be an opportunity to reduce their exposure to toxins and chemicals.

Whether it's choosing organic and natural materials for clothing and toys, opting for eco-friendly diapers and skincare products, or embracing sustainable feeding and hygiene practices, non toxic baby care is about making thoughtful choices that benefit both your child and the world they live in. By incorporating eco conscious principles into your baby care routine, you can provide a safe, healthy and nurturing environment for your little one.

Natural and Non Toxic Skincare Products for Baby

Choosing natural and non toxic skincare products for your baby is essential for their delicate skin and overall health.

Organic and Natural Oils
Look for skincare products containing organic oils such as coconut oil, olive oil, jojoba oil or almond oil. These oils are nourishing, moisturising and are gentle on baby's sensitive skin.

Shea Butter
Shea butter is a natural moisturiser that helps soothe and protect baby's skin. It is rich in vitamins and antioxidants, making it an excellent choice for dry or irritated skin.

Calendula
Calendula is a gentle and soothing herb known for its anti-inflammatory and healing properties. Skincare products containing calendula extract or oil

can help calm and comfort baby's skin.

Chamomile:

Chamomile is another soothing herb that can help reduce inflammation and irritation. Look for skincare products containing chamomile extract or oil to help soothe baby's skin.

Non Toxic Formulations:

Choose skincare products that are hypoallergenic and free from common allergens such as fragrances, dyes and harsh chemicals. This reduces the risk of irritation and allergic reactions in your baby's sensitive skin.

Always read the ingredient list carefully and look for certifications such as USDA Organic or EWG Verified to ensure the products meet high safety and purity standards.

Homemade Baby Care Recipes

Creating homemade non toxic baby care products is a wonderful way to ensure that your little one is exposed to only gentle and natural ingredients.

DIY Baby Wipes

Ingredients:

1 cup distilled water

1 tablespoon liquid castile soap

1 tablespoon fractionated coconut oil

1 drop organic lavender essential oil (optional)

Instructions:

Mix all ingredients together in a bowl.

Cut an entire paper towel roll in half with a sharp knife.

Place one half of the paper towel roll in an airtight container.

Pour the liquid mixture over the paper towels until they are fully saturated.

Seal container securely and use wipes as needed.

DIY Baby Powder

Ingredients:

1/2 cup arrowroot powder or non-gmo cornstarch

1 tablespoon finely ground oats (optional)

1 drop organic lavender or chamomile essential oil (optional)

Instructions:

Mix arrowroot powder or cornstarch with finely ground oats in a bowl.

Add essential oil drops if desired and mix well.

Store in a clean, airtight container.

DIY Baby Oil

Ingredients:

1/2 cup organic sweet almond oil

1/4 cup organic jojoba oil

1/4 cup fractionated coconut oil

5 drops organic chamomile or lavender essential oil (optional)

Instructions:

Mix all oils together in a clean bottle or jar.

Add essential oil drops if desired and shake well to combine.

Use as a gentle moisturiser for baby's skin after bath time.

DIY Baby Bath Soak:

Ingredients:

1/4 cup finely ground organic oats

1/4 cup dried organic chamomile flowers 1/4 cup dried organic lavender buds

Instructions:

Combine all ingredients in a muslin bag or cheesecloth pouch.

Place the bag in the bathtub as it fills with warm water.

Allow the bag to steep in the water for a few minutes before bathing baby.

DIY Baby Lotion

Ingredients:

1/2 cup organic coconut oil

1/4 cup organic shea butter

1/4 cup organic cocoa butter

1/4 cup organic sweet almond oil or jojoba oil

1 tablespoon beeswax pellets (for thicker lotion)

1 teaspoon vitamin E oil (natural preservative)

1 drop organic lavender or chamomile essential oil

Instructions:

Melt the Ingredients:

In a double boiler, combine the coconut oil, shea butter, cocoa butter, sweet almond oil (or jojoba oil), and beeswax pellets.

Stir occasionally until all the ingredients are completely melted and combined.

Remove the mixture from heat and allow it to cool slightly.

Add the vitamin E oil and a few drops of essential oil (if

using) and stir well to combine. Whip the Lotion:

Allow the mixture to cool to room temperature.

You can speed up this process by placing the bowl in the refrigerator for about 15-20 minutes.

Once the mixture starts to solidify but is still soft, whip it using a whisk or hand mixer until it becomes light and fluffy.

Store the Lotion:

Transfer the whipped lotion into clean glass jars or lotion containers.

Store in a cool, dry place. The lotion should last for several months, especially if you included vitamin E oil.

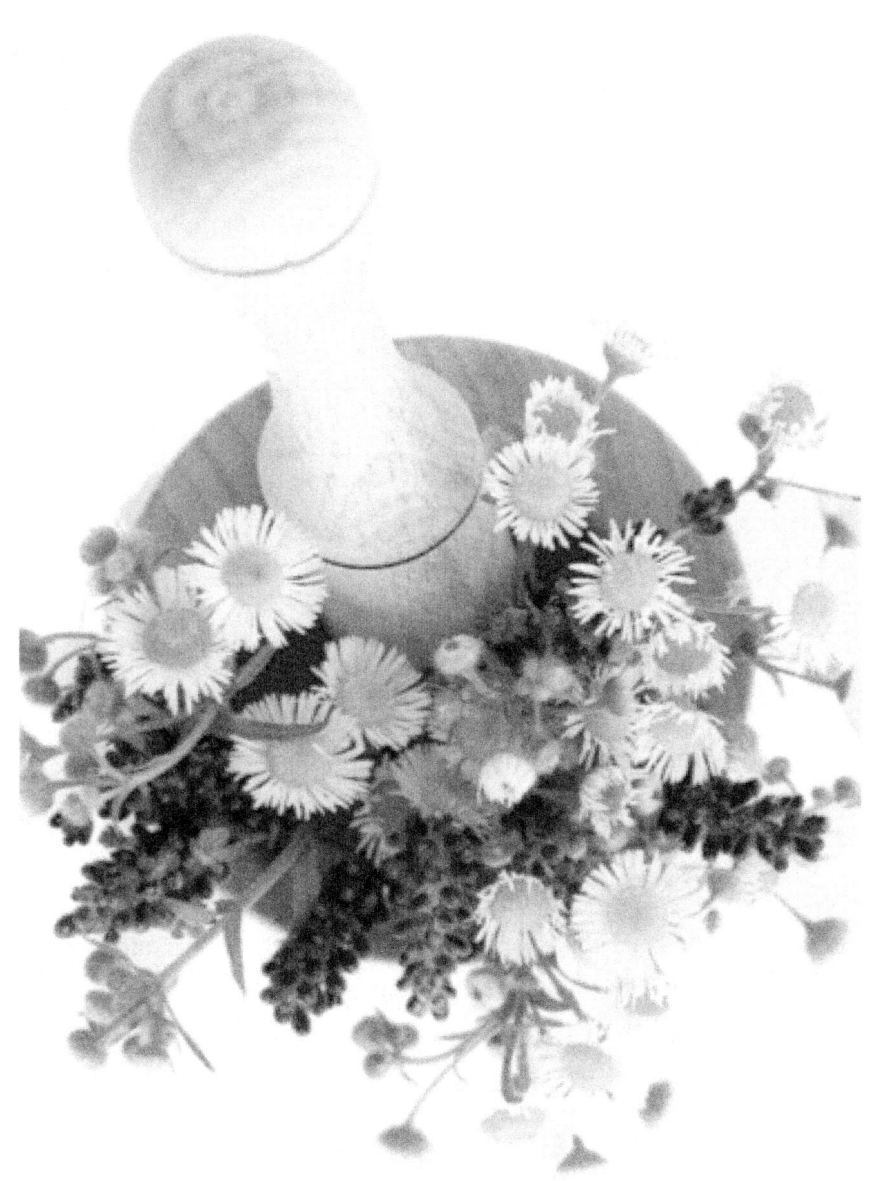

Sustainable Bath Time Practices

Sustainable bath time practices for your baby can help reduce waste, conserve water and minimise your environmental footprint.

Use Natural and Chemical-Free Products

Choose natural and chemical-free baby wash, shampoo and skincare products made with gentle, plant-based ingredients. Look for products that are free from synthetic fragrances, dyes and harsh chemicals to minimise exposure to harmful substances.

Conserve Water

Fill the bathtub with only as much water as necessary to comfortably bathe your baby. Consider using a bathtub insert or a small basin to reduce the amount of water needed for each bath. Turn off the tap while washing and rinsing your baby to conserve water.

Bathe Less Frequently

Babies don't need daily baths, especially newborns. Instead, aim for 2-3 baths per week to keep your baby clean without over-washing. Spot clean areas like the face, neck and diaper area between baths as needed.

Use Washcloths or Reusable Wipes

Instead of disposable wipes which often contain chemicals and fragrances, use soft washcloths or reusable cloth wipes made from organic cotton or bamboo. Wash and reuse these wipes to reduce waste and avoid the use of single-use disposable products.

Choose Non Toxic Bath Toys

Choose bath toys made from non toxic materials such as natural rubber, food-grade silicone or sustainably sourced wood. Avoid plastic toys that may contain harmful chemicals like BPA or PVC.

Dry Naturally

Allow your baby to air dry or gently pat them dry with a soft, organic cotton towel after the bath.

Repurpose Bath Towels

Once your baby outgrows their bath towels, re-purpose them as cleaning rags or donate them to animal shelters for use as bedding.

Consider Showering Together

As your baby grows older, consider showering together as a family to save water and bond with your little one. Always ensure the water temperature is safe and comfortable for your baby.

By incorporating these sustainable bath time practices into your routine, you can provide a safe and non toxic nurturing bathing experience for your baby.

DIY Non Toxic Bath Products for Baby

Castile Soap Baby Wash

Ingredients

1/2 cup liquid castile soap (unscented or mild baby formula) 1/4 cup distilled water

1 tablespoon vegetable glycerin

1 tablespoon fractionated coconut oil

5 drops of organic lavender or chamomile essential oil (optional, for fragrance)

Instructions

In a clean container, combine the liquid castile soap, distilled water, vegetable glycerin, and fractionated coconut oil.

Add 5 drops of essential oil if you'd like to add a gentle fragrance to the wash.

Stir the ingredients together until well combined. Transfer the mixture to a clean, empty bottle with a pump or flip-top cap for easy dispensing.

Shake well before each use. Use as you would any commercial baby wash, lathering onto your baby's skin and rinsing thoroughly with warm water.

As with any new product, it's a good idea to do a patch test on a small area of your baby's skin before regular use to check for any adverse reactions.

Oatmeal and Honey Baby Bath Soak

Ingredients

1/2 cup finely ground oats

1/4 cup dried organic chamomile flowers or lavender buds 2 tablespoons raw honey

1 tablespoon fractionated coconut oil

Muslin bag or cheesecloth pouch (optional)

Instructions

In a clean bowl, mix together the finely ground oats, dried chamomile flowers or lavender buds, raw honey, and fractionated coconut oil until well combined.

If using, place the mixture into a muslin bag or cheesecloth pouch and tie securely to create a tea bag-like pouch.

Hang the pouch under the tap/faucet as you fill the baby's bath with warm water. Alternatively, you can place the pouch directly into the bath water.

Allow the bath soak to steep for a few minutes to release the soothing properties of the oats and herbs. Gently squeeze the pouch to release more of the oatmeal and herbal goodness into the water. Remove the pouch from the bath water before placing your baby in the tub. Bathe your baby as usual, using the water infused with the oatmeal and herbal mixture to cleanse their skin.

These DIY non toxic bath wash recipes are gentle and nourishing for your baby's delicate skin, providing a soothing and safe bath time experience. As with any new product, it's a good idea to do a patch test on a small area of your baby's skin before regular use to check for any adverse reactions.

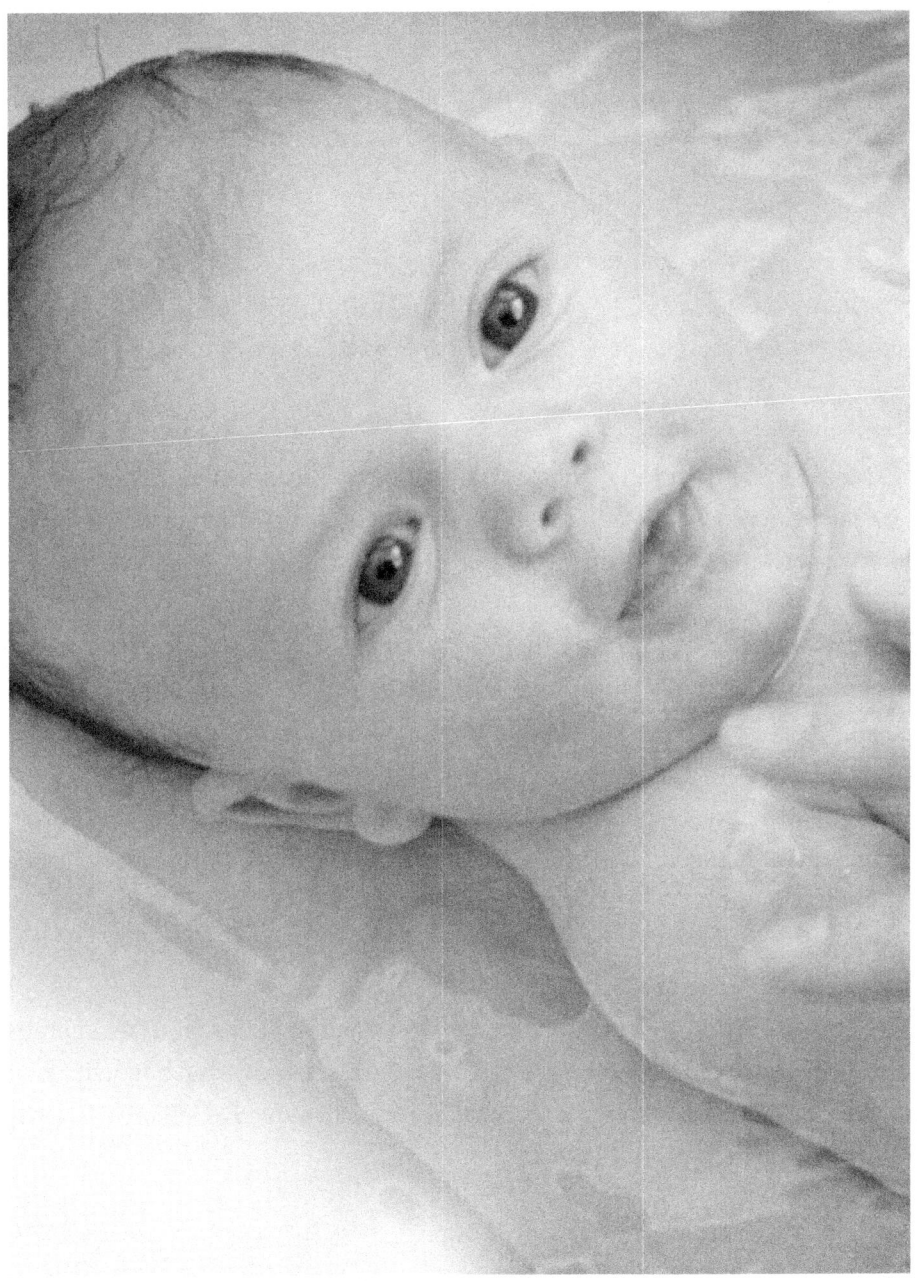

Eco Friendly Playroom Design

Designing an eco friendly and toxin free playroom for your baby is a wonderful way to create a safe, nurturing and sustainable environment where they can learn, explore and grow.

Choose Non Toxic Paint

Use zero-VOC or low-VOC paint for the walls and furniture to minimise indoor air pollution and reduce exposure to harmful chemicals.

Natural Flooring

Choose natural flooring materials such as bamboo, cork or hardwood, which are durable, renewable and free from toxic chemicals which can be found in many synthetic flooring options.

Natural Light

Maximise natural light in the playroom by incorporating large windows, skylights and sheer curtains to allow plenty of sunlight to flood the space.

Energy-Efficient Lighting

Install dimmer switches or use lamps with adjustable brightness to create a cosy and comfortable ambiance for playtime.

Sustainable Furniture

Select eco-friendly furniture made from sustainable materials such as bamboo, reclaimed wood or FSC- certified (Forest Stewardship Council) wood. Look for furniture with non toxic finishes and adhesives to ensure a healthy indoor environment.

Modular and Multi-Functional Design

Choose modular furniture pieces that can be easily reconfigured to adapt to your baby's changing needs as they grow. Incorporate multi-functional furniture such as storage ottomans, convertible cribs and play tables with built-in storage to maximise space and minimise clutter.

Natural Textiles

Use organic cotton, hemp or bamboo textiles for rugs, curtains and upholstery to create a soft and cosy environment for play. These natural fibres are breathable, hypoallergenic and free from the harmful chemicals found in synthetic fabrics.

Toy Rotation System

Implement a toy rotation system to minimise toy clutter and reduce waste. Store toys in baskets or bins made from natural materials such as seagrass or jute, and rotate them periodically to keep playtime fresh and exciting.

Greenery and Indoor Plants

Bring nature indoors by incorporating potted plants and indoor greenery into the playroom. Not only do plants improve air quality and promote relaxation, but they also provide opportunities for sensory exploration and learning about the natural world.

Recycled and Upcycled Decor

Decorate the playroom with eco friendly decor items made from recycled or upcycled materials, such as reclaimed wood shelves, vintage artwork or handmade crafts. Get creative and re-purpose items from around your home to add a personal touch to the space.

Air Purifying Plants

Choosing air purifying and non toxic indoor plants for your baby's playroom is a great way to improve indoor air quality and create a healthy environment.

Spider Plant (Chlorophytum comosum)

Spider plants are known for their air purifying abilities. They are easy to care for and can tolerate a wide range of light conditions, making them ideal for indoor spaces.

Snake Plant (Sansevieria trifasciata)

Snake plants are excellent air purifiers. They have a unique upright growth habit and can thrive in low light conditions, making them perfect for a baby's nursery or playroom.

Peace Lily (Spathiphyllum spp.)

Peace lilies are effective at removing toxins from the air. They produce beautiful white flowers and prefer indirect light, making them a lovely addition to a playroom or nursery.

Rubber Plant (Ficus elastica):

Rubber plants are hardy and easy to care for, making them suitable for beginners. They are excellent air purifiers and can tolerate low light conditions, making them perfect for indoor spaces with limited sunlight.

Parlor Palm (Chamaedorea elegans)

Parlor palms are compact and easy to care for, making them suitable for small spaces like playrooms and nurseries.

Boston Fern (Nephrolepis exaltata)

Boston ferns are known for their air purifying properties. They thrive in high humidity environments and prefer indirect light, making them ideal for bathrooms or humid playrooms.

Areca Palm (Dypsis lutescens)

Areca palms are excellent at removing indoor air pollutants. They require bright, indirect light and regular watering to thrive, making them a great choice for well-lit playrooms.

Bamboo Palm (Chamaedorea seifrizii)

Bamboo palms are effective at filtering indoor air. They prefer bright, indirect light and regular watering, making them suitable for playrooms and nurseries with ample sunlight.

When selecting indoor plants for your baby's playroom, be sure to choose varieties that are safe and non toxic. All the above plants are listed as safe for babies, but for added caution keep them out of reach of little hands and mouths and be mindful of any potential choking hazards such as small leaves or berries.

With proper care and placement, indoor plants can enhance the air quality and ambiance of your baby's play and sleeping space, while providing a safe and natural environment for them to rest, explore and grow.

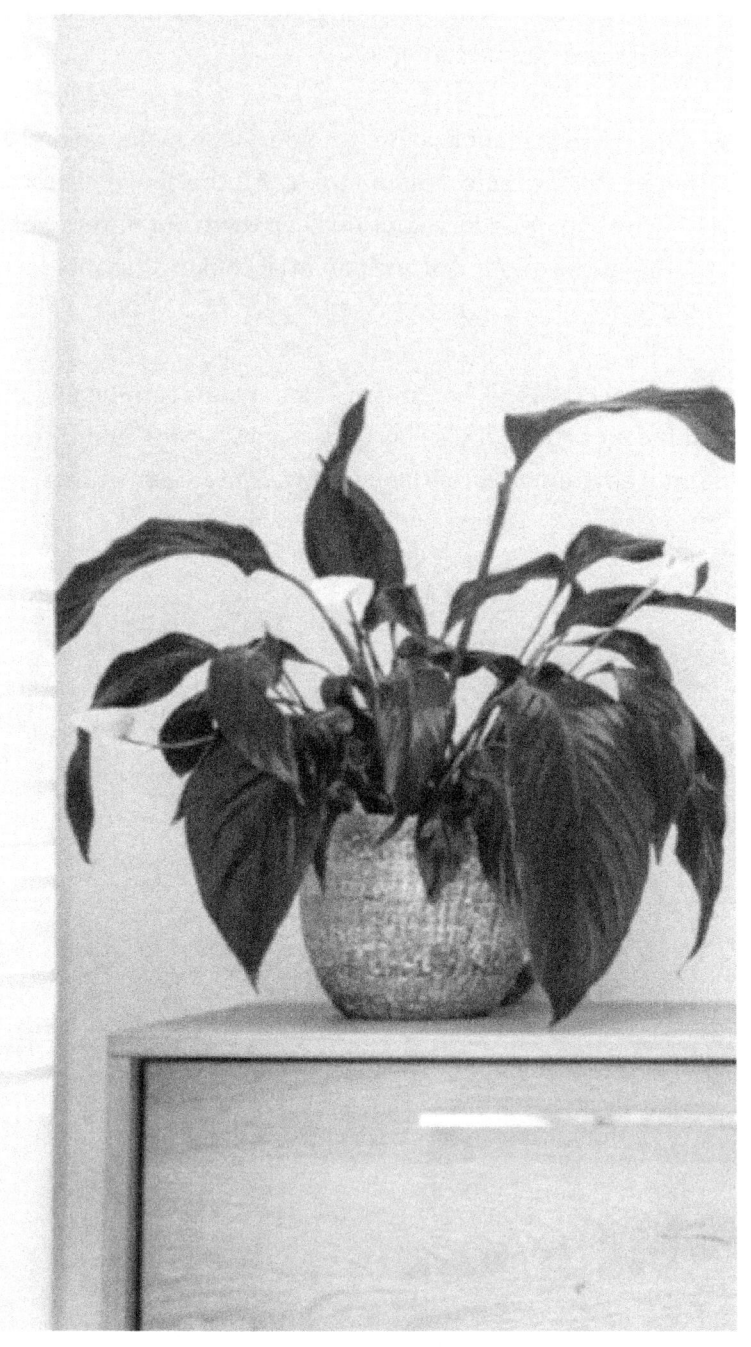

Outdoor Nature Play and Exploration

Outdoor exploration play and activities for babies provide wonderful opportunities for sensory stimulation, physical development and connection with nature.

Nature Walks

Take your baby for leisurely strolls in nature, such as parks, gardens or nature trails. Point out different sights and sounds, touch textures like tree bark or leaves, and let your baby explore the natural world at their own pace.

Tummy Time in the Grass

Lay a soft blanket or mat on the grass and let your baby enjoy tummy time outdoors. The grass provides a different sensory experience and encourages your baby to engage their muscles while observing their surrounding area.

Sensory Play with Natural Materials

Set up a sensory bin or tray filled with natural materials such as sand, water, rocks, pinecones or leaves. Let your baby explore and manipulate the materials with their hands and senses, encouraging curiosity and discovery.

Garden Exploration

If you have a garden or outdoor space, involve your toddler baby in simple gardening activities such as digging in the soil, watering plants with a small watering can, or picking ripe fruits or vegetables. Engage their senses as they discover the sights, smells and textures of the garden.

Outdoor Music and Movement

Set up a designated outdoor play area with soft mats or cushions where your baby can crawl, roll, or practice standing and walking. Play music or sing songs outdoors and encourage your baby to move or dance to the rhythm.

Nature Scavenger Hunt

Create a simple nature scavenger hunt for your older baby by searching for specific items such as flowers, birds, insects or different types of leaves. Use pictures or simple descriptions to guide your baby's exploration and encourage observation skills.

Outdoor Water Play

On warm days, set up a shallow water play area with a small tub or basin filled with water and safe water toys. Let your baby splash, pour and explore the water with cups, spoons and containers, providing a refreshing and stimulating sensory experience.

Picnic in the Park

Pack a picnic blanket and some baby-friendly snacks and head to the park for a relaxed outdoor meal. Let your baby explore the surroundings, watch other children play and enjoy the sights and sounds of nature.

Animal Watching

Visit a local petting zoo, farm or nature reserve where your baby can observe animals in their natural habitats. Point out different animals, make animal sounds and talk about their characteristics and behaviours.

Outdoor Storytime

Set up a cosy outdoor reading nook with a blanket or cushions and read books aloud to your baby. Choose stories with nature themes or colourful illustrations that capture your baby's attention and spark their imagination.

Remember to prioritise safety during outdoor playtime by providing adequate sun protection, staying hydrated, closely monitoring your baby around any type of water activity, and watching for any signs of discomfort or fatigue.

Health Benefits of Grounding for Babies

Grounding, also known as earthing, is the practice of connecting with the Earth's surface by walking barefoot, sitting or lying down directly on the ground. While research on grounding specifically for babies is limited, there are several potential health benefits associated with grounding.

Improved Sleep

Grounding has been shown to help regulate circadian rhythms and improve sleep quality by syncing the body's internal clock with natural light-dark cycles. Babies who are grounded may experience more restful sleep patterns.

Reduced Inflammation

Grounding has been found to have anti-inflammatory effects by neutralising free radicals and reducing oxidative stress. This can potentially help alleviate symptoms of inflammation-related conditions, such as eczema or asthma, in babies with these health concerns.

Stress Reduction

Grounding has been associated with decreased levels of cortisol, the stress hormone, in the body. Babies who are grounded may experience reduced stress and anxiety levels, leading to a greater sense of calm and wellbeing.

Enhanced Immunity

Some studies suggest that grounding may support immune function by reducing inflammation and promoting overall health and vitality. Babies who spend time connecting with the earth may experience a boost in their immune system's ability to fight off infections and illness.

Improved Mood and Emotional Wellbeing

Grounding has been linked to improvements in mood, emotional stability and overall mental health. Babies who are grounded may exhibit greater happiness, contentment and emotional resilience.

Pain Relief

Grounding has been shown to have analgesic effects, reducing pain and discomfort associated with various conditions. Babies who are grounded may gain relief from teething pain, colic or general discomfort.

Better Balance and Coordination

Grounding involves direct contact with the earth's surface, which can stimulate the body's proprioceptive system and improve balance and coordination skills. Babies who spend time grounded may develop these motor skills more quickly and effectively.

Enhanced Connection to Nature

Grounding encourages a deeper connection to the natural world, fostering a sense of appreciation, wonder and reverence for the Earth and its ecosystems. Babies who are grounded from an early age often develop a lifelong affinity for nature and outdoor activities.

Always prioritise safety and supervision when practicing grounding with infants, ensuring that they are comfortable and protected from potential hazards while connecting with the ground.

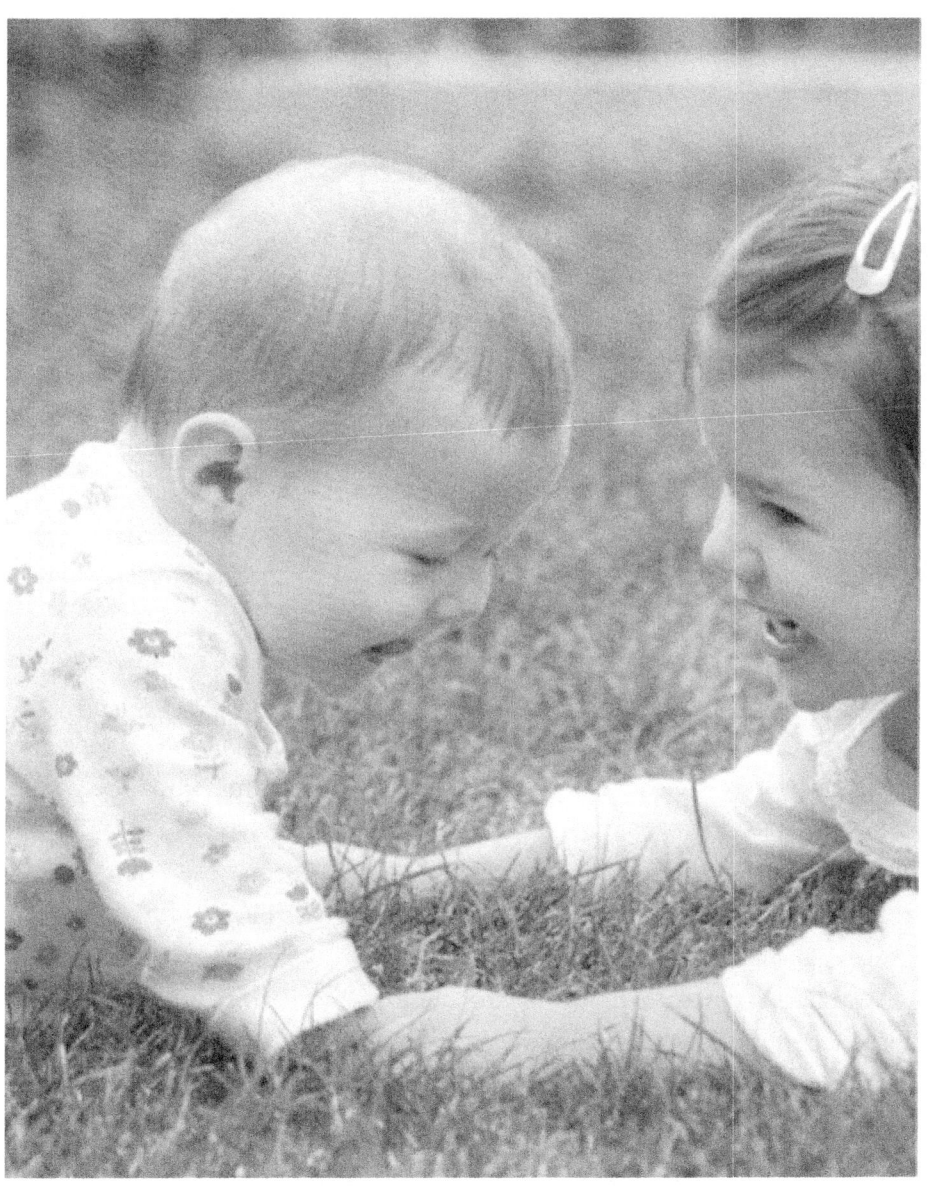

Eco Conscious Travel with a Baby

Eco conscious travel with a baby involves thoughtful planning and mindful preparation.

Plan Ahead

Research eco conscious and baby-friendly options for accommodation, activities and transportation before you go.

Sustainable Accommodations

Green Hotels: Stay in hotels with eco-friendly practices, such as non-smoking rooms, use of non toxic cleaning products, energy-efficient lighting and water-saving measures.

Vacation Rentals: Consider renting a home or apartment, which often uses fewer resources than large hotels.

Eco Lodges: These accommodations are designed to have minimal environmental impact.

Camping and Glamping: Eco friendly campsites and glamping sites can be a great way to stay close to nature as a family with minimal impact.

Eco Friendly Activities

Nature-Based Activities: Enjoy outdoor activities like hiking, swimming and exploring nature trails.

Local Experiences: Support local economies by visiting farmers' markets, local shops and community events.

Educational Tours: Participate in eco-tours that focus on conservation and sustainability.

Food and Feeding

Breastfeeding: If possible, breastfeeding is the most easy and sustainable feeding option.

Homemade Baby Food: Prepare your own baby food using local, organic ingredients. Store it in reusable, food-grade silicone containers.

Eco Travel Accommodation with a Baby

The eco travel industry has made significant strides in accommodating families with babies. Whether you choose to stay at a large resort, a boutique hotel or an eco-lodge, you can find many options that cater specifically to the needs of eco-conscious families with babies.

Baby Equipment: Choose accommodations that offer essential baby equipment such as cribs or bassinets, high chairs, changing tables and baby baths for an easier travelling experience. Enquire in advance if baby carriers, car seats, strollers or pushbikes with baby seats are available for guest use.

Room Essentials: Always check if the rooms are baby-proofed with outlet covers, secured furniture for baby's that are at the crawling or pulling-themselves-up stage, and there are no small, easily swallowable objects for curious hands and mouths.

Accommodations with kitchenettes, which include sterilisers and bottle warmers, make travelling with a baby, and especially feeding time, much more enjoyable. Soundproofed or quiet rooms help your baby to sleep undisturbed. Check if the accommodation includes a washer/dryer for baby's clothing, or a guest laundry service.

Eco Friendly Travel Activities With a Baby

Travelling with a baby offers a unique opportunity to engage in eco friendly activities that are generally outdoors and gentle on the environment.

Nature Walks and Hikes
   Short and Easy Trails: Choose trails that are stroller-friendly or baby carrier-friendly. Nature walks provide fresh air and gentle exercise for both you and your baby.
   Wildlife Watching: Look for areas with opportunities to observe birds, butterflies or other wildlife.

Botanical Gardens and Parks

Botanical Gardens: These are perfect for leisurely walks with a stroller. Babies can enjoy the sights and sounds of various plants, flowers and insects.

Public Parks: Enjoy picnics and playtime in open, green spaces. Many parks also have playgrounds suitable for young children.

Beach Days

Eco-Friendly Beaches: Visit beaches known for their clean and eco friendly practices. Bring reusable containers and utensils for snacks and meals.

Shallow Waters and Tide Pools: Shallow water areas are generally safer for babies to play and explore. Tide pools can offer gentle, educational experiences with marine life.

Sustainable Farms and Markets

Farm Visits: Organic and sustainable farms often offer tours where you can see animals and learn about eco-friendly farming practices. These can be educational and enjoyable for babies and parents alike.

Local Markets: Visit farmers' markets to enjoy fresh, locally-sourced foods, while supporting local farmers and producers.

Eco Friendly Zoos and Aquariums

Accredited Zoos and Aquariums: Only choose to visit zoos and aquariums with a strong focus on conservation and animal welfare. Most public zoos have baby-friendly facilities and educational programs.

Interactive Exhibits: Many zoos and aquariums have touch tanks or safe, interactive exhibits suitable for young children.

Bicycle Rides

Bike Rentals: Many destinations offer bicycle rentals with baby seats or trailers. It's a sustainable way to explore local areas while enjoying the outdoors.

Scenic Bike Paths: Choose bike riding routes that are safe, smooth and scenic, avoiding busy roads with heavy air pollution.

Educational Visits

Eco-Centres and Nature Reserves: Many nature centres and reserves offer educational programs and exhibits about local ecology and conservation efforts.

Museums with Eco-Exhibits: Some museums have sections dedicated to the environment, sustainability, and nature, often with interactive displays suitable for young children.

Outdoor Picnics

Reusable Supplies: Choose locations with beautiful natural surroundings where you can relax and your baby can play. Bring your own reusable picnic supplies to reduce waste.

Eco-Friendly Snacks: Pack organic, locally-sourced snacks and drinks.

Community Activities

Local Environmental Events: Participate in local eco friendly events such as beach clean-ups or tree planting. These are often community-oriented and family-friendly.

Cultural Experiences: Engage with local traditions and practices that emphasise sustainability and respect for nature.

By incorporating these eco friendly activities into your travel plans, you can enjoy meaningful, low-impact experiences that are enjoyable for you and your baby, while also fostering a connection with nature and supporting sustainable practices.

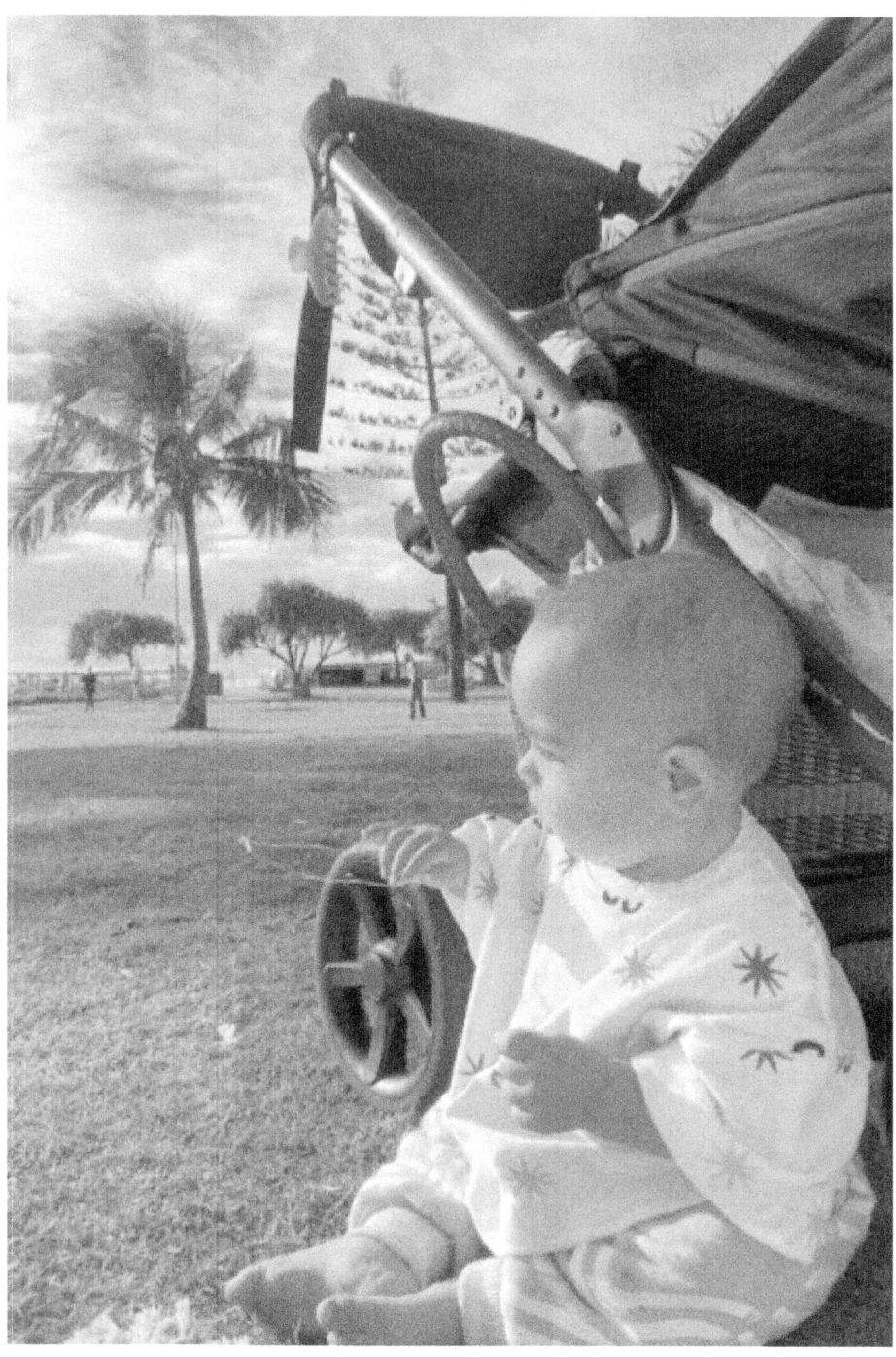

Pack Light and Smart

Make a checklist to ensure you bring all your baby's essentials, reducing the need to buy disposable products during your trip. Pack only what is necessary to make travel easier. Bring reusable wipes, bottles and snack containers to reduce waste.

Cloth Diapers: These can be washed and reused, reducing waste. Don't forget your eco friendly diaper bag.

Biodegradable Disposable Diapers: For convenience when out hiking or walking with baby, use biodegradable disposable diapers to reduce your environmental impact.

Reusable Wipes: Cloth wipes are a sustainable alternative to disposable ones and can be washed and reused.

Silicone Bibs: Easy to clean and reusable.

Bottles and Utensils: Use stainless steel or glass bottles and reusable silicone utensils.

Reusable Snack Containers: Bring snacks in reusable silicone or fabric pouches, or stainless steel containers.

Eco-Friendly Baby Items: Choose items made from sustainable materials, such as organic cotton clothing and bamboo blankets.

Multipurpose Items: Select multi-functional gear to minimise the amount you need to bring. Muslin blankets made from organic cotton can serve as swaddles, nursing covers, light blankets or stroller covers.

Second-Hand and Borrowed Items: Consider borrowing or renting baby gear at your destination to reduce the need for new purchases.

Green Practices During Travel

- Use natural and organic products for you and your baby's skin care and health needs.
- Ensure all eco friendly gear meets safety standards to keep your baby comfortable and secure during travel.
- Turn off lights, heating and air conditioning when not in use. Choose accommodations with non toxic products and energy-efficient appliances.
- Avoid single-use plastics and bring reusable bags, bottles and utensils.
- Buy local produce and dine at restaurants that source their ingredients locally and sustainably.
- Traveling during off-peak times can reduce your environmental impact, is usually more cost effective, and with less crowds, makes for a more relaxed trip.
- Use the trip as an opportunity to teach older children about the importance of sustainability.
- Participate in local conservation projects or clean-up activities as a family.

Final Words......

Nurturing a safe, healthy and non toxic home environment for your baby is highly beneficial and recommended for their overall wellbeing.

By incorporating non toxic and eco friendly practices into every aspect of your family life, from creating an eco-friendly nursery to making homemade baby food and DIY baby products, you are providing a healthier home for your child, while significantly reducing your environmental footprint.

Engaging in DIY arts and crafts fosters creativity and sustainability, while choosing non toxic floor and wall coverings ensures a safe and clean space for your baby to play and grow. Embracing eco-conscious travel practices allows you to explore the world sustainably, teaching your child the importance of caring for the environment from an early age.

By adopting these holistic approaches and eco friendly ways of living, you are not only protecting your family's health but also instilling values of sustainability and responsibility that will last a lifetime.

Together, we can create a brighter, greener, healthier future for our children, our children's children, and the world they grow up in.

About the Author

Donna Attard, an Australian mother and grandmother, is filled with wisdom and knowledge in the realms of holistic wellbeing, eco conscious and non toxic living and natural pregnancy and parenting.

As the visionary founder of EcoandOrganic.com, Donna has established a nurturing sanctuary for families seeking understanding, guidance and support. Through her books, audios and courses, she offers a wealth of resources and insights, empowering families to embrace natural and non toxic approaches to pregnancy, parenting and life in general.

In addition to her written works, Donna has curated a transformative collection of meditation and self-hypnosis audios meticulously crafted to foster wellbeing during pregnancy, parenting and childhood. These soothing audios serve as invaluable tools for those seeking to cultivate inner peace and relaxation.

Donna's unwavering dedication to promoting holistic wellness and eco friendly living continues to inspire and uplift countless of individuals around the globe. She has touched the lives of many, with a legacy of love, empowerment and conscious living.

Resources

Website: EcoandOrganic.com

Eco Friendly and Healthy Living books
    Non Toxic Living at Home book bundle
    How to Make Your Home Healthy & Eco Friendly
    Make Your Own Green Cleaning Products
    Stylish & Sustainable: Ethical Fashion for the Eco Chic
    Disclosure 101: Healthy Living Secrets Hidden in Plain Sight
    Sun, Sand & Sustainability: A Guide for the Eco Conscious on the Gold Coast

Adult Guided Meditations
    Pool of Tranquillity Meditation
    Relaxation for Beginners Meditation

Children's Books
    Rocket Ride to Outer Space: Encourages Self Confidence
    The Peaceful Fairy Pond: Relieves Stress and Anxiety

Children's Guided Meditations
    Magical Butterfly Meditation
    Guardian Angel Meditation
    Peaceful Dolphins Meditation

Organic Essential Oils
    EcoandOrganic.com

Non Toxic & Sustainable Products for Babies

Strollers & Stroller Gear
    Era - Reversible Stroller. All terrain, city style.
    Bumbleride - Organic Cotton Stroller Insert
    Apple Park - White Jellyfish Stroller Toy

Baby's Nursery
    Organic Crib Mattress
    Blaynk - Organic Cotton Baby Swaddle

Baby Personal Care
    2 in 1 Baby Body Wash and Shampoo
    Organic Tapioca Starch Baby Powd

Oral Health
    Finger Toothbrush
    Children's Tooth Gel 6+ months
    Camilia Teething Relief, 1+ Month

Baby
    100% Cotton Onesie
    Organic Cotton Socks
    Organic Muslin Burp Cloths

Baby Toys
    Organic Knit Bunny
    100% Natural Rubber Duck
    Natural Rubber Eco-Teether
    Organic Kozy Koala
    Sustainable Rubberwood Tug Boat
    Wee Gallery Inc - Bamboo Nesting Hedgehog

References

Books

Smith, R., & Lourie, B. (2009). *Slow death by rubber duck: The secret danger of everyday things.* Knopf Canada.

Wentz, M., & Wentz, D. (2011). *The healthy home: Simple truths to protect your family from hidden household dangers.* Vanguard Press.

Gavigan, C. (2008). *Healthy child, healthy world: Creating a cleaner, greener, safer home.* Dutton.

Landrigan, P. J., & Needleman, H. (2001). *Raising healthy children in a toxic world: 101 smart solutions for every family.* Rodale Press.

McDonough, W., & Braungart, M. (2002). *Cradle to cradle: Remaking the way we make things.* North Point Press.

Marriott, S. (2008). *Green baby: The practical guide to raising a happy, healthy, eco-friendly baby.* Duncan Baird Publishers.

Colborn, T., Dumanoski, D., & Myers, J. P. (1997). *Our stolen future: How we are threatening our fertility, intelligence, and survival.* Penguin Books.

Websites and Eco Organisations

Environmental Working Group. (n.d.). *Research and reports.* https://www.ewg.org/

Natural Resources Defense Council. (n.d.). *Toxics and health.* https://www.nrdc.org/

Global Organic Textile Standard. (n.d.). *Global Organic Textile Standard (GOTS).* https://www.global-standard.org

Healthy Child Healthy World. (n.d.). *Creating a cleaner, greener, safer home.* Environmental Working Group. https://www.healthychild.org

American Lung Association. (n.d.). *Indoor air quality.* https://www.lung.org

EcoCert. (n.d.). *Certifications for organic and eco-friendly products.* https://www.ecocert.com

Campaign for Safe Cosmetics. (n.d.). *Research on toxins in cosmetics.* https://www.safecosmetics.org

Green America. (n.d.). *Green living resources.* https://www.greenamerica.org

International Journal of Environmental Research and Public Health. (n.d.). *Research on environmental toxins and health risks.* https://www.mdpi.com/journal/ijerph

Pediatric Environmental Health Specialty Units. (n.d.). *Environmental health risks for children.* https://www.pehsu.net

Environmental Health Perspectives. (n.d.). *Journal articles on environmental health.* https://ehp.niehs.nih.gov

Organic Consumers Association. (n.d.). *Research on organic standards and toxins in consumer products.* https://www.organicconsumers.org

Environmental and Parenting Journals

Journal of Exposure Science and Environmental Epidemiology. *Articles on VOCs, air quality, and environmental exposures affecting children.* https://www.nature.com/jes/

International Journal of Environmental Research and Public Health. *Covers various environmental toxins and their impact on human health, particularly children.* https://www.mdpi.com/journal/ijerph

Environmental Health Perspectives (EHP). *Peer-reviewed journal with a focus on environmental health risks, including toxins in homes.* https://ehp.niehs.nih.gov/

Journal of Toxicology and Environmental Health (2024). *Research on the effects of environmental toxins on child development.* https://www.tandfonline.com/toc/uteh20/current

Sustainable Living Blogs & Resources

The Minimalist Mom – https://www.theminimalistmom.com

Mama Natural – https://www.mamanatural.com

Green Child Magazine – https://www.greenchildmagazine.com

EcoParent Magazine – https://www.ecoparent.ca

Mindful Momma – https://mindfulmomma.com

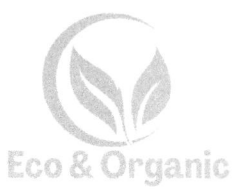

Eco and Organic Store Product Page

Full range of Toxin Free Living, Eco Parenting and Children's books and meditations. EcoandOrganic.com

Social Media
　IG: @eco_and_organic
　Fb: Eco and Organic Living

Printed in Great Britain
by Amazon